Nutritional Evaluation

OF

SPROUTS

AND

GRASSES

Viktoras P. Kulvinskas, M.S.
former Director of Research
Hippocrates Health Institute, Boston

OMANGO D' PRESS
P.O. BOX 255, WETHERSFIELD, CONN. 06109

Contents

INTRODUCTION

This is the most informative and instructional book on sprouts that I have read. It helps me to understand why it is helpful to sprout seeds and grains. It lists many vitamins, minerals and essential nutrients which are commonly recognized. It describes a special test, the chromatogram, which shows there are properties in "live" foods which are not measured in milligrams and international units. It gives many interesting facts gleaned from an extensive bibliography.

I am responsible for my own health, as each person is for his. It is time for each of us to think about the forms of treatment which work with the natural forces for health in the body. One of the best health measures and treatments is raw food and especially sprouts.

Because sprouts are easy to grow, because they are available throughout the year, because they are economical, saving us money and time in buying and preparing foods, and most important because they are so full of nutrients and energy, the use of sprouts is increasing by leaps and bounds each year.

The people in our nation and our world can be healthier and happier by eating more whole foods.

Good Sprouting!!

Ruth Rogers, M.D.

Preface

The Sprouts Are Coming! **No, the sprouts are already here.** Once they were relatively unknown outside of health food circles. Now sprouts can be found virtually everywhere. They are used by catering services, airlines, hospitals, old age homes, schools, steakhouse salad bars, etc. They are sold everywhere: in health food stores, in major supermarket chains, even at open-air vegetable stands. I have seen alfalfa sprouts, mung bean sprouts and cress sprouts proudly displayed in stores that had not sold them previously because of a lack in public demand. But those days are gone — people know about and want sprouts. Sprouts have achieved such public acclaim that the Wall Street Journal investigated sprouts and consequently released a long article discussing and supporting the claims made about their nutritional value.

Sprouts are being discussed in print and are being explored by many different journals and researchers. Based on information I have received from a nationally prominent researcher, I'll predict that a cure for cancer will be found, using a diet consisting primarily of sprouts and live foods. Many researchers are exploring solutions to cancer through diet and other "wholistic" measures. In a Houston, Texas hospital, studies by Dr. Chiu Lai show success in controlling and correcting several types of cancer cells using the juice of sprouted wheat. The government, too, is interested in the potential of wheatgrass juice. The government has financed an experiment designed to test the effect of wheatgrass juice on cancer cells in rats.

Current cancer treatment is not a pleasant or successful experience. The chance to be healed without the suffering required by standard treatment (chemotherapy and radiation) is such a dream to those afflicted with cancer, that to speak of such a possibility without research and documentation would be unjust. To show further proof, I'll mention the research of an American Nobel Prize winner. He has researched the effect of sprout diets on cancer for two years, and has found that sprouts have a very positive effect on animals with cancer. His findings will be published toward the end of 1978. This study will be followed up with a study on human beings organized by the Ortho-molecular Research Institute. Starting in May, human volunteers, thoroughly checked before and after, will go on a 30-day diet of raw food, sprouts and wheatgrass juice.

Live food therapy and research is not confined to the United States. Dr. Ann Wigmore of the Hippocrates Health Institute has started a 4-month project in India to research the therapeutic value of wheatgrass juice against cancer and other forms of degenerative diseases. In conjunction with ALL of India Wheat Grass Research Center, using over 30 doctors and hundreds of patients, wheatgrass therapy will be explored, documented and most important of all, utilized in a hospital setting.

We are fortunate to have received and accepted the concept that health needs to be approached wholistically. The research into wholistic methods has placed a divine light in the pathway to health. Health is so dependent on lifestyle, diet and thought, that any improvement in one of these areas reflects directly in a person's health. Wholistic is an idea born in universal truth. Proof of this statement lies in the universal success and its universal applicability. Everyday I receive letters from doctors turning toward wholistic methods. My mail is filled with letters of gratitude, personal testimonials and inspirational notes of rejuvenation. We are making great gains in helping ourselves. But as significant as our gains are, we should all realize that this is only the beginning. We have just begun to use the light within, and I know that we shall never lose sight of the light. The light will help us learn things that we didn't even know existed.

I am very grateful to be a part of this enlightening process. Today, the reasons for our existence are being explored and discussed in many ways. We have journeyed into the frontier of total consciousness as we learn how to balance our various levels of being. Many teachers are here to make available the means to physical, mental, emotional and spiritual well-being. I know some of these teachers. I feel privileged to have met, studied with, assisted, and carried on in my own way the light of these teachers and their teachings.

I remember my first experience along the path. I became a vegetarian and lost one hundred pounds of unhealthy tissue. After a few years of detoxification, my weight stabilized at 135 lbs. Along with my change in physical appearance came a change in my outlook on life. I started to look for the meaning of life in my own being. These were days of excitement that resulted from self-exploration and pioneering into new ways of thinking. It was at this time that I encountered the force within me. I was moved by the force of my true self, away from the security of college life, where I taught computer consultation, into the unknown, unheralded field of consciousness.

Today, it is considered fashionable to leave middle class ways in order to explore the meaning of life. Ten years ago, when I started my adventure, self exploration was thought of in negative terms. I felt alone in response to the ridicule and consequent loss of friends. Yet, this separation was the bridge to my inner world. The force within became a solid foundation to guide and energize my activities.

I was guided to Dr. Ann Wigmore of Rising Sun Christianity. In the safety of her farm and mansion, I labored and learned the crafts of survival. Here we explored the healing properties of sprouts and grasses. Eventually we founded the Hippocrates Health Institute to advance and utilize therapy using sprouts and grasses.

The diet at Hippocrates evolved to the point where we discarded all usage of cooked foods. We used only a live food diet consisting primarily of sprouts, green juices, fermented seed milks, baby greens, vegetables, sea vegetables and seasonal fruits. Each year we had thousands of resident guests who enjoyed the taste and healing properties of our special diet. Hippocrates is known throughout the world, its theories nurtured by Dr. Ann's 20 years of service along with my 10 years. Recently, I saw a beautiful example of live food's international appeal. A store in Hawaii was selling sunflower seed yogurt, 3-day instant saurkraut, sunflower greens, buckwheat lettuce and wheatgrass. Additionally, a group of 17 people in Austin, Texas, ran a raw food restaurant — The Greenlight Juice Bar — based on a model described in my book, "Survival Into The 21st Century."

Live foods are accepted as healing agents today and are used at over 30 health resorts as therapeutic tools. Recognition of the importance of live foods in academics is occurring, too. Soon, a 4-year naturopathic college, sponsored by the Foundation for Natural Living, will open in Northern California. The college will advocate a diet centered on sprouts.

I have compiled a directory, listing over 3000 subjects related to live foods and New Age events. The directory's purpose is to make available the "tools" necessary in undertaking a journey into health. I have devoted a lot of myself to finding and defining correct steps along the path to health. I would like all of you to help join in this search. Help yourself and help each other in the work of healing. Let me suggest a simple but very effective way to start that healing process.

Every week, set aside one day. On this one day eat or drink nothing save green juice. Then each month, set aside an entire weekend. Set up your weekend as a special 3-day holiday. Make it an excursion into prayers, self-exploration, consciousness expansion and fasting. Each day of the weekend drink juices and other purification methods that are described in "Survival Into The 21st Century." You will improve your health markedly by using this simple and inexpensive formula.

Diet does not only affect our physical being. Evidence shows that the mind, body and soul are an interrelated unit. As the food becomes purer, the energy of both the food, body and mind increases. A purer diet leads directly to increased consciousness. This has been repeatedly demonstrated using kirlian photography and experiments in ESP. Also, there are records of happiness and bliss induced by grass juices and hunger as well as diet-related improvements in concentration, creativity, and relaxation.

The earth is a paradise, and it will be realized when we stop abusing nature, the mother of paradise. Earth is the base of mother nature and earth is part of our being. The first step toward achieving paradise is to till, plant and grow the earth that lies within. From castles of light shall the light go forth.

Yours lovingly,

INTRODUCTION

WANTED: A live vegetable that will grow in any climate, rival meat in nutritional value (and tomatoes in vitamin C), matures in three to five days, may be planted any day of the year, requires neither soil nor sunshine, has no waste, can be eaten raw.

Dr. Clive McCay of Cornell University composed this ad which would perplex all of us if it were carried in the daily papers. The Chinese, centuries ago, captured the "good guy: soybean" and have been "fletcherizing" it ever since.

This band of Robin Hood type outlaws, headed by the soybeans, includes such big-timers as garbanzo, untamed peanut, Ho Chia Mung, as well as the lesser stature of wheat, alfie, and the radical radish. Matter of fact, the qualifications to join this underground (some aboveground) brotherhood, is to be an organic, sproutable seed.

If the sprouts ever group forces on a large scale with the creeping weeds and the biblical grasses, and start infiltrating the supermarkets and sneaking into the salad bowls of outstanding members of our society, they will cause the most radical revolution in our diet and destroy many of our highly respected utensils, as well as our institutions. You will see hospitals eliminated by the explosives of live food, drug factories and research firms will become inhabited by wise spiders and their networks of cobwebs, insurance will be re-

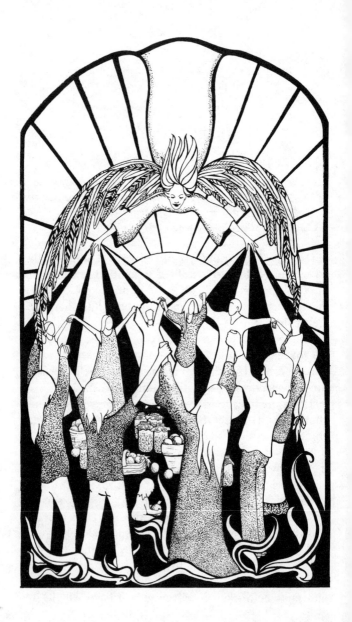

placed by honesty, old age homes will be converted to tennis courts, butcher knives will become museum pieces, vivisection and animal experimentation will be considered sadism. During the transition, those who have not yet discarded their greed will be trying to make a profit by selling to the receptive plans for cenverting stoves into refrigerators and cooking pots into indoor garden containers.

SPROUTS IN HISTORY

These lowly little warriors will lead civilization into a new world of humanity and the era of fruitarianism. And we shall return to the natural law: *"And the fruit thereof shall be for meat, and the leaf thereof for medicine."* (Ezekiel 47:12).

Sprouts have a history as old as civilized man's use of seed. One of the earliest references to sprouting comes in the Book of Daniel, Chapter 1, 10-20:

> *"And the prince of eunuchs said unto Daniel, I fear my Lord the king, who had appointed your meat and your drink: for why he should see your faces worse liking than the children which are of your sort? Then shall ye make me endanger my head.*
>
> *"Then said Daniel to Melzar, whom the prince of eunuchs had set over Daniel, Hannaniah, Mishael, and Azariah,*
>
> *"Prove thy servants, I beseech thee, ten days; and let them give us pulses to eat, and water to drink.*
>
> *"Then let our countenance be looked upon before thee, and the countenance of the children that eat of the portion of the King's meat: and as thou seest, deal with thy servants.*
>
> *"So he consented in this matter, and proved them ten days.*
>
> *"And at the end of ten days their countenances ap-*

> peared fairer and fatter in flesh than all the children
> which did eat the portion of the king's meat . . .
>
> "And in all matters of wisdom and understanding
> that the King inquired of them, he found them ten
> times better than all the magicians and astrologers
> that were in all his realm."

It took only ten days to produce miraculous results. Today it would take longer. Daniel and his comrades ate the pulses (sprouted seeds) in the tradition of Jesus. Professor Edmon Szekely translates from ancient documents found in the Vatican Library: *"Moisten your wheat, that the angel of water may enter it. Then set it in the air, that the angel of air may embrace it. And leave it from morning to evening beneath the sun, that the angel of sunshine may descend upon it."* This process is known as sprouting. (1)

Sprouts are one of the essential ingredients in the diet of the Hunzas, who are noted for an extremely long life span and unsurpassed health. Such foods provide them nutrients during the cold winters in the Himalayan Mountains. All people of Asia are familiar with sprouts. Germinated or otherwise, the soybean is used by the Orientals as their main source of quality protein. Most Americans taste soy or mung sprouts for the first time in Chinese restaurants and wonder where such funny looking food grows.

LOVE LIFE OF A SPROUT

All changes have an electromagnetic nature. One might say that every sprout is a miniature transmitter-receiver station that reacts to the emotional level of its immediate surroundings. For centuries, it has been suspected that growing plants do more than just sit in the soil and soak up the sun. The possibility that or-

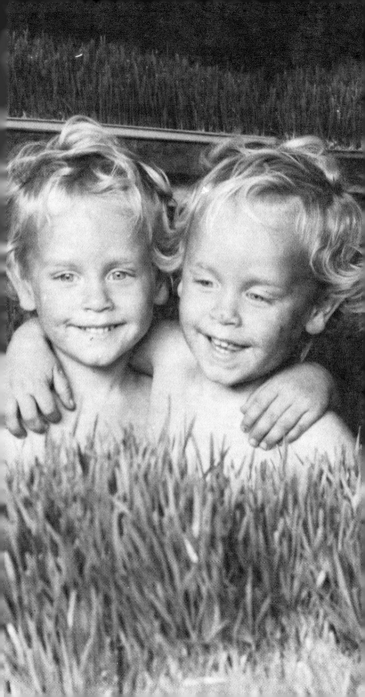

dinary vegetation is capable of "consciousness" goes as far back as the Egyptians. Jesus is recorded as speaking to an unproductive fig tree to cause it to wither.

Sprouts are very sensitive to electro-magnetic field orientation. There is an optimal growth position, a change from this orientation will slow the growth (111). Thus, far better results are attained by growing them in buckets with holes. The buckets are not moved, and are watered from top.

However, the most important influence comes from the sproutarian. From the philosophy and practical experience at Findhorn comes these words (111):

> *"The most important contribution that man or woman can make to a garden—even more important than water or compost—is the radiation one puts into the soil while cultivating it, such as love . . . plants are constantly being affected by radiation from the earth itself and from the cosmos, which were more fundamental than chemical elements or microbiotic organisms, radiations that are subject fundamentally to the mind of humans. Individuals appear to have the role of a demigod; by cooperating with nature one might find no limit to what one can achieve on this planet . . . Divina had managed to get into direct contact with the devas or angelic creatures who control the nature spirits that are said by clairvoyants to be everywhere at work nurturing plant life."*

There are ways of concentrating the cosmic and magnetic energy for increased rate of growth. Studies have been done to see the effect of pyramid power on sprouts (112):

> *1. In all cases, the pyramid treated plants grew 2 to 3 times as fast as the controls, were more healthy and lasted longer after the harvest.*
> *2. The pyramid grown sprouts lasted over a week*

without spoilage after the harvest. The controls lasted 24 to 36 hours before spoilage.

3. The sprouts in the pyramid dehydrated slightly but did not decay and resumed normal growth when watering was resumed. The controls developed odors and died.

Rodale (Prevention) has shown that one can attract cosmic radiation by surrounding plants with copper wire, chicken fence wire mesh, or metallic objects. The overall effect is two to three times faster growth and higher germination rate.

Dr. Robert Jerome, a botanist at the University of Mexico, directs E.S.P. messages to plants in his laboratory. By feeding positive emotions toward plants, he is able to make them grow rapidly. By daily applications of hate, he is able to cause plants to wither and die in five weeks, although they receive proper care of soil, water and sunlight.

Minister Franklin Loehr (50), a chemist, is convinced that a prayed-over seed grows faster than one not so treated. He and his researchers have experimented now with 20,000 seeds and have to their satisfaction demonstrated that prayer, when done right, visibly, objectively, and repeatedly, affects germination and growth.

Thoughts of love and well-being are states of consciousness: they affect everything—other people, animals, plants and minerals. One should strive to reach a higher state of awareness instead of negating the life force of other beings. When you sprout, if you discover that the seeds grow slowly, it might not be a problem of technique—it might be your state of consciousness. The sprouts are listening, brothers and sisters!

SEA SPROUTS SAVE SCURVY

The fact that germinated legumes will prevent and cure scurvy has been known since the 18th century. Charles Curtis, a surgeon in the British Navy, wrote the passage quoted below in a book published in 1807. Curtis was drawing on the experience of a "Mr. Young of the Navy" who wrote a report on scurvy in 1782 (118):

> "Nothing more is necessary for the cure of this disease in any situation where there is tolerably pure air than—not dead and dried, but fresh vegetable diet, greens or roots, in sufficient quantity. To be sure, we cannot have a kitchen garden at sea, and only a short and scanty crop of greens can be raised on board ship; but beans and peas, and barley and other seeds brought under the malting or vegetative process, are converted into the state of a growing plant, with the vital principle in full activity throughout the germ and pulp. If eaten in this state without any sort of preparation, except that of separating and rejecting the husk, they cannot fail to supply what is wanted for the cure of scurvy, viz., fresh vegetable chyle."

Charles Curtis went on to express a preference for "gram", an East Indian grain, chiefly used in the feeding of horses (presumably mung or chick peas).

A review (2) of related literature shows that as early as 1912, Holst and Frolich proved experimentally that vegetables of high antiscorbutic potency became useless for the prevention of scurvy when dried and made suitable for military supply. In 1912 the use of germinated seeds was proposed as a solution to the problem. The menace of scurvy to British and Indian troops in Mesopotamia during 1915 and 1916 attracted the attention of Lister Institute to the earlier work, resulting in an extensive study by Chick and Delf which led to the discovery that dry peas and lentils, when germinated, had considerable "antiscorbutic stuff—."

Germinated broad beans were used by Wiltshire (1918) to cure cases of scurvy in the First World War; and an outbreak in a famine area in India in 1940 was brought under control by the distribution of sprouted chick peas.

In a review (18) of literature on ascorbic acid Chattapadhya and Benerjee of President College observed that the ascorbic acid reaches its maximum on the third day of germination. A parallel activity seems to be occurring, so that in mung, as well as in other pulses studied, during the course of the germination on the fourth day the dehydro-ascorbic acid value is maximum (6). Total soy bean ascorbic acid increased roughly 5.5 times in 48 hours, 6 to 7 times in 54 hours and slightly more in 72 hours. Biotin (37) tripled in 5 days of germination.

A 100-gram serving (31), about a quarter pound of sprouted soybeans or sprouted peas raw, as shown in the table below, would provide approximately the following values of ascorbic acid, depending on the time of harvest. On the sixth day you would be eating ascorbic acid content in the bean in the same high concentration found in lime juice. One cup of 6 day old soy sprout can supply 1.5 times the minimum daily requirements of vitamin C. One cup of mung bean sprout contains even higher amounts.

ASCORBIC ACID			
Hrs.	*mg/100g*	*Hrs.*	*mg/100g*
0	0	72	71.8
24	8.2	96	82.9
48	27.2	120	102.8

Seeds

The seed is a storehouse of food energy intended for early growth and development of the new plant. The chemical changes that occur in the sprouting seed activate a powerful enzyme factory, never to be surpassed at a later stage of growth. The sprouts are predigested foods. The rich enzyme concentration can lead to heightened enzyme activity in your own body metabolism, thus leading to regeneration of the bloodstream.

DORMANCY AND LIFE-SPAN OF SEEDS

"Diaspore dormancy has at least three functions: (1) immediate germination must be prevented even when circumstances are optimal so as to avoid exposure of the seedling to an unfavourable period (e.g., winter), which is sure to follow; (2) the unfavourable period has to be survived; and (3) the various dispersing agents must be given time to act. Accordingly, the wide variation in diaspore longevity can be appreciated only by linking it with the various dispersal mechanisms employed, as well as with the climate and its seasonal changes. Thus, the downy seeds of willows, blown up and down rivers in early summer with a chance of quick establishment on newly exposed sandbars, have a life-span of only one week. Tropical rain forest trees frequently have seeds of low life expectancy also. Intermediate are seeds of sugarcane, tea, and coco palm, among others, with life-spans of up to a year. Mimosa glomerata *seeds in the herbarium of the Museum National d'Histoire Naturelle in Paris were found viable after 221 years. In general viability is better retained in air of low moisture content. Some seeds, however, remain viable under water—those of certain rush* (Juncus) *species and* Sium cicutaefolium *for at least seven years. Salt water*

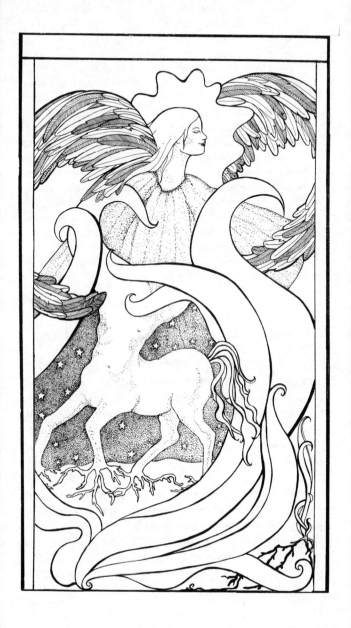

can be tolerated for years by the pebble-like but float-ing seeds of Caesalpinia (Guilandina) bonduc and C. bonducella, *species that, in consequence, possess an almost pantropical distribution. Seeds of the sacred lotus* (Nelumbo nucifera) *found in a peat deposit in Manchuria and estimated by radioactive-carbon dating to be 1,400 (± 400) years old, rapidly germinated and subsequently produced flowering plants) when the seeds were filed to permit water entry. In 1967 seeds of the arctic tundra lupine* (Lupinus arcticus)̄, *found in a frozen lemming burrow with animal remains established to be at least 10,000 years old, germinated within 48 hours when returned to favourable condi-tions. The problem of differential seed viability has been approached experimentally by various workers, one of whom buried 20 species of common Michigan weed seeds, mixed with sand, in inverted open-mouthed bottles for periodic inspection. After 80 years, three species still had viable seeds." (127)*

SOAKED SEEDS NUTRITIONAL VALUES

The dry seed is characterized by a remarkably low metabolic rate, but even moistening of seed triggers tremendous changes. Professors A.M. Mayer and A. Poljakoff-Mayber (p. 101) of the Botany Department, Hebrew University, Jerusalem, describes (3) the pro-cess: *"As soon as the seed is hydrated, very marked changes in composition in its various parts occur. These changes occur even when seed is placed in water without any nutrients, and in complete absence of assimilation. The chemical changes which occur are complex in nature. They consist of three main types: the breakdown of certain materials in the seed, the transport of materials from one part of the seed to another, especially from the endosperm to the embryo or from the cotyledons to the growing part, and lastly*

*the synthesis of new materials from the breakdown
products formed. The only substances normally taken
up by the seeds during germination are water and
oxygen."*

The high activity that goes on in the seed was illus-
trated in a study by Baily (21) of the University of
Minnesota. He showed that in Zea mays seeds the out-
put of carbon dioxide rose from .7 mg. per hundred
grams dry weight during twenty hours, at 11 percent
moisture, to about 60 mg. when moisture reached 18
percent, or a total increase of 87 times the original.
Similar increases can be observed for rice, wheat and
others.

After soaking the seed in distilled water, do not feel
that the soak water can be discarded without a second
thought. On May 10, 1970, Ann Wigmore received a
communication from Harvey C. Lisk (119) who
showed the composition of the soak water through
quality tests utilizing paper chromatography. Lentils,
alfalfa, wheat and mung were soaked individually.
Then a mixture of all four seeds were soaked collec-
tively for 12 hours. At the end of the period the
mineral content of water had been raised as follows:
Wheat .30%, Lentils .35%, Mung Beans .55%, Alfalfa 2.0% and the mixture .40%. Furthermore, the
test showed the soak water to be especially high in
quality factors of minerals, vitamins, enzymes and
amino acids. The live mineral value added to the distilled water is quite low, but it stops the leeching effect
of distilled water.

ENZYME PROCESS

Sprouts are noted for their high enzyme activity
never to be surpassed at later stage of maturity (7).

Among the essential enzymes are amylase, which acts upon starches; protease to digest protein; lipase, a fat-splitting protein; coagulase, coagulate milk or clot blood; emulsin, which acts upon sugar; invertase which converts cane sugars into dextrose.

Some of the orthodox nutritionists maintain that enzymes from vegetation are unnecessary because the human body makes its own and that they will have no favorable effect on metabolism. However, other experts present substantial proof that enzymes are very important in human diet (128, 129). New evidence indicates that both vitamins and minerals must be bound up in enzyme complex (130), such as is the case in chelated minerals, in order to be beneficially effective.

Tom Spies, M.D., strongly emphasizes the need of natural foods in ones diet for optimal health (131):

> *"The respiration and growth of cells involve the synthesis of complex substances from simpler chemical compounds. By means of substances called enzymes, the cells are able to perform these functions without increased temperature and pressure.* Enzymes *are* catalysts *produced by living cells from combinations of organic substances, including the vitamins. These enzymes retain activity even when separated from a living cell. When a dietary deficiency of vitamins has existed over a long period of time, a biochemical lesion develops in the cell, often severe enough to cause functional disturbances. If the deficiency is not corrected, these disturbances become more widespread and eventually give rise to an infinite variety* of symptoms *forming a* complex clinical *picture. Finally, severe or persistent alterations lead to structural changes in the tissue, and ultimately the diagnostic lesions of a deficiency disease are likely to appear. The* complexity *of the subject is greatly increased by the fact that the several groups of the various* vitamins usually occur together in nature, *and the* failure *to provide* one *usually results in*

failure *to* provide many. *Then, one has arising from a dietary fault* innumerable, vague, indefinite symptoms *coming from cells affected because a number of* catalysts *are* not working efficiently."

"Often isolation and synthesis of a new vitamin shake the structure of medical theory to its foundation, and usually bring new hope to the sick and afflicted. Unfortunately, the application of these findings with vigor and enthusiasm has led to thinking too much *in* terms of isolated vitamin deficiencies, *although every method of study has indicated the predominance of* mixed rather than single deficiency of elements *essential for life and well-being."*

STARCH METABOLISM

Wheat is one of the staple foods of the world. In 3 days of sprouting, the weight doubles and a very sweet tang is introduced. Much of the original starch has been converted to natural sugars. When complemented with chick peas and a little seakelp, it makes a very satisfying meal, giving you a complete protein, and all of the other needed nutrients.

In a Japanese publication, a study reveals that sucrose is the main component of the endosperm of cereals before germination. However, in wheat and buckwheat, glucose was found at a level equal to that of sucrose. Other sugars—stachyose, maltose and raffinose—were minor components. Sucrose decreased to 50-80 per cent of the original level, and glucose increased markedly during 4 to 6 days of germination. Glucose and sucrose were the main components of shoots and roots of the germinated cereals.

In wheat (7, 8) steeped for two days, the starch diminished, resulting in a twofold increase in sucrose

21

content, maltose sixtyfold, gluco-difructose fourfold, and reffinose threefold, thus making sprouted wheat a quick energy food.

Professor Yocum grew wheat in soil and analyzed the composition of both the entire seed or seedling and, after separation into different organs was possible, also the composition of the endosperm, root and plumule. Table 1, shows some of the results obtained. It should be noted that starch decreased continuously in the endosperm as well as the whole plant. Dextrins also disappeared from the endosperm. Fats also decreased during the first few days, but later fats became reformed in predigested states. (42)

The change in the starch of barley during sprouting have been studied in detail because of its importance in the malting process (3, 148):

> *"Glucose and fructose rise very considerably up to six days germination at 21°C and then begin to fall again . . . Maltose rose from about 1 mg per gram dry seeds to more than 55 mg after 7 days of germination (representing 5500% increase). Almost as great an increase occurred in oligosaccharides"*— *Raffinose and maltose increased five fold by seventh day.*

Grain becomes less mucous-forming after sprouting. Linke and Miller (29) 1959, noted a marked decrease in glutamate, which virtually disappeared from excised wheat germ. In a much earlier publication, Kozmina (30) noted that up to the 4th day of sprouting there is only a small decrease of gluten but it undergoes marked qualitative changes, becoming crumbly.

Young and Varner (11), showed that amylase activity increased sevenfold in the first six days of germinating peas. Amylase breaks most of the starch down to simple sugars. In soybean much of the starch is converted to simple carbohydrates. Lee et al of Seoul

TABLE 1

CHANGES IN COMPOSITION OF WHEAT SEEDS DURING
GERMINATION AND GROWTH

The results are given as weight of substances in mg per
100 seeds or parts of seedlings.

(Compiled from Yocum, 1925)

Time in days	Plant Part	Dry weight	Ether extract lipids	Total sugar	Dextrin	Starch
0	Original Seed	2685	66.9	53.9	43.5	1781.0
1	Seed	2708	63.1	44.7	82.0	1621.3
2	Seed	2593	57.6	137.2	111.0	1079.0
3	Seed	2544	51.0	121.4	81.3	1343.5
6	Seedling	2476	45.9	465.8	120.5	472.1
9	Seedling	2383	95.3	208.9	86.5	117.5
12	Seedling	2031	94.7	37.1	19.9	20.2
3	Plumule	110	2.1	9.2	3.3	2.6
6	Plumule	383	8.7	20.4	9.6	2.9
9	Plumule	875	54.8	26.5	11.7	7.0
12	Plumule	1054	68.3	4.1	3.0	0
3	Root	103	2.6	6.3	2.5	1.5
6	Root	286	6.1	14.8	5.2	0.6
9	Root	469	10.7	15.5	6.8	1.5
12	Root	691	10.2	12.5	7.8	2.3
3	Remaining Seed (endosperm)	2332	46.3	105.9	75.4	1339.5
6	(endosperm)	1807	31.2	430.7	105.7	468.0
9	(endosperm)	839	29.7	167.0	60.1	109.0
12	(endosperm)	287	16.3	20.5	8.9	17.9

University showed (31) that sucrose, stachyose and raffinose are the main sugars in soybean; germination converts the latter two into glucose and fructose-sugars that are present in fruit.

FAT METABOLISM

Fats and oils are converted by the action of lipases. Drs. Mayer and Poljakoff-Mayber state (3): "Normally neither of the breakdown products of hydrolysis of lipids accumulates in the seed . . . it seems to become part of the general carbohydrate pool present in the seed . . . In many seeds disappearance of fats is accompanied by the appearance of carbohydrates." The elimination of complex fat structures improves tremendously the digestibility of sprouts over seeds.

The detailed course of fat metabolism has been traced by Hardman and Crombie (12) and Boatman and Crombie (13) in a variety of seeds. In Citrullus vulgaris there is a rapid break-down of lipids both in the cotyledons (seed leaf) and in the rest of the seed. Yamada (14) observed that lipase activity in the endosperm of the castor bean increased by twenty-fold in the first 80 hours of germination. Brown et al (124) observed the crude fat of soybean decrease and free fatty acids increase. White noted a significant drop in the total saturated fatty acid content (125).

A well known nutritionist, C. Ellwood (26) states:

> "Experiments show that in sunflower and pumpkin seeds the fats are converted into carbohydrates. In legumes, the fats take a quick nose dive the first five days but gradually return to their original amounts . . . in the wheat seedlings the fat increases all the way through the sprouting period."

In a later study, 1953, Chattopadhya and Benerjee (19) show that there is a significant increase in choline, a lipotrophic agent that controls fat metabolism. All legumes are high in it as compared to grains. Mung, which has three times the value found in wheat or rice, showed choline increase from 205 mg. per 100 grams to a value of 260 after 4 days of growth. This was a 27 percent increase. During the same time, wheat showed a 30 percent increase.

When an experimental diet fails to supply the essential fatty acids (EFA), the animal develops scally skin condition, sores, poor growth and premature death (149).

Dr. Pottinger maintained health, good growth rate and reproductive capacity of animals for several generations during the course of the experiment (26) while feeding the animals with sprouts.

Dr. C. F. Schnabel (115) reported a twelve week experiment with guinea pigs. On a sole diet of dried, organic grass and water, the animals maintained an excellent growth rate. The coat was shiny, no skin problems. If animals were maintained on a vegetable diet consisting of carrot, lettuce, cabbage and/or canned spinach, the animals showed a gradual weight decline, skin and structural disorders, as well as death by the 7th week. However, once grass was reintroduced the animals maintained a normal growth rate.

These two experiments point out that the sprouts and/or grasses can supply the essential fatty acids. The fats are either in the food, or else the diet contains precursors from which the body can build E.F.A.

For a more detailed study of the subject, one can read the 1977 revised version of another book (49) by the author.

PROTEIN METABOLISM

According to some authorities (3), there is usually little change in the total nitrogen content of the seed or seedling during germination, although slight losses may occur especially due to the leeching out of nitrogen substances. Mayer and Poljakoff-Mayber (3) concluded from many studies that during germination in the dark, proteins are broken down into amino acids.

Other researchers are discovering that in the germination process plants synthesize some new protein (119) from carbohydrates and fats (121). The material presented by Nandi (123) shows that in the seeds studied there was an increase in the total amount of all amino acids. The total protein content per mung bean seed rose on the average from 25% in dry seed to 37% in dried sprout. Similar increase was observed in the sprouted soybean (122).

Virtanen et al (16) showed that during germination of pea seed there occurs a rapid synthesis of new amino acids. Pfeiffer (126) of Bio-Dynamics Laboratories made similar observations about wheat, where lysine, one of the essential amino acids, appeared on the seventh day of sprouting.

The following tables show the daily changes in amino acids which occur during germination (126):

What occurs during germination is a reduction in protein concentration as in the case of soybean (9), from 34.1 to 6.2 percent, and for mung bean from 24.2 to 3.8 percent. The reason for a reduction to one-sixth of its previous concentration, is due to an approximate six-fold increase in moisture.

If you have a well-balanced amino acid composition in a seed, you can anticipate the same balance in the sprout, except less concentrated. Soybean is a good example (6). Such decrease in protein concentration

26

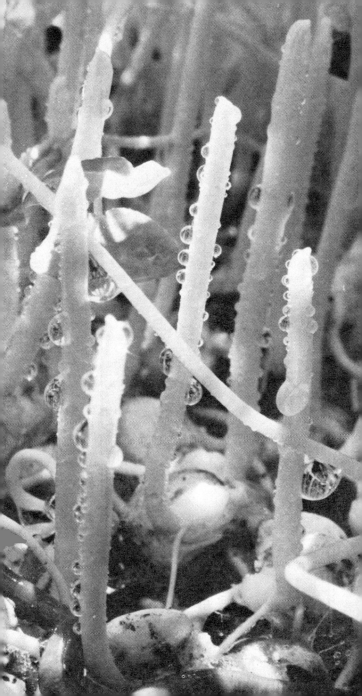

Days after germination

Barley:	4th			5th			6th			7th		
	O	F	C	O	F	C	O	F	C	O	F	C
Arginine	7	9	9	7	6	7	7	6	7	7	6	7
Aspartic Acid	3	2	2	5	5	10	5	6	10	5	5	5
Glutamic Acid	2.5	3	8	2.5	2.5	6	5	5	8	5	8	8
Leucine	0.2	0.2	1	0.2	0.8	1	0.2	0.8	1	0.2	0.5	0.2
Lysine	1.5	1.5	1.5	0	0	0	0	0	0	0	0	0
Methionine	1.5	2	3	2	2	3	2	2	2	2	2	2.5
Threonine	2	2	5	5	10	10	5	8	10	5	5	7
Tyrosine	0.5	1	3	0	0	1	0	0	0	0	0	0
Valine	0.1	0.1	0.7	0.1	0.5	0.7	0.1	0.5	0.7	0.5	0.05	0.7

O—Control, tap water. A sprout.   F—Formula of mineral supplement product   C—Extract from compost

TABLE 2

The figures in the following tables indicate content in microgram per gram of leaf:

Days after germination

Wheat:	5th			6th			7th			9th		
	O	F	C	O	F	C	O	F	C	O	F	C
Arginine	18	40	40	20	20	40	9	7	9	9	6	18
Aspartic Acid	15	20	25	25	25	40	20	14	40	30	35	50
Glutamic Acid	8	12	18	12	18	25	6	8	15	5	6	18
Leucine	1	2	5	2.5	2	10	1	1	5	2.5	2.5	5
Lysine	0	0	0	0	0	0	0	0	0	2	1.5	3
Methionine	3	3	5	3.5	5	10	3.5	2	4	2	3	3
Threonine	2	5	3	3	5	10	4	2	7	2	1.5	5
Tyrosine	0	1	1	0	1	1.5	1	1.5	3	1.5	1	2
Valine	0.7	2	5	0.8	0.9	1	0.7	0.1	1	0.6	0.6	1

O—Control, tap water. A sprout.   F—Formula of mineral supplement product   C—Extract from compost

		Days after germination										
		4th			5th			6th			7th	
Oats:	O	F	C	O	F	C	O	F	C	O	F	C
Arginine	9	9	18	40	40	40	9	9	18	18	18	18
Aspartic Acid	20	20	25	25	20	20	5	10	20	10	10	20
Glutamic Acid	4	5	5	8	8	8	5	5	8	16	16	18
Leucine	1	1	2.5	2.5	5	6	2	2.5	5	1	1	2.5
Lysine	0	0	0	0	0	0	0	0	1.5	0	0	0
Methionine	2	2	2	2	2	2	3	3.5	5	2	3	5
Threonine	4.5	4.5	4.5	4.5	10	20	3	5	10	10	5	5
Tyrosine	2	2	4.5	1	1	1	tr.	tr.	tr.	1	1	1
Valine	0.7	0.7	0.7	5	5	5	0.7	1	1	0.7	0.9	0.8

O—Control, tap water. A—sprout.   F—Formula of mineral supplement product   C—Extract from compost

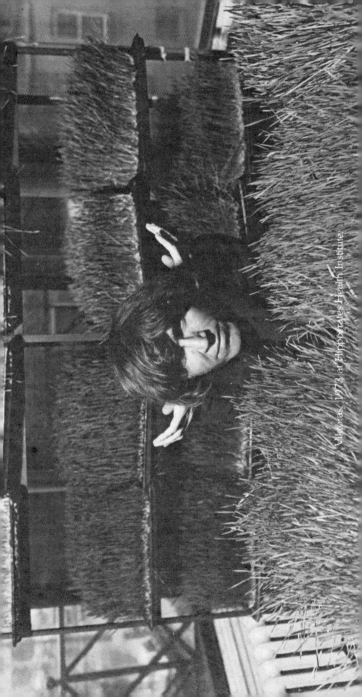

is highly beneficial in terms of human fruitarian physiology. Furthermore, the protein is in the form of amino acids and enzymes, without the associated metabolic uric acid. Because sprouts are predigested food, they have a higher biological efficiency value than whole seeds, raw or cooked. Less food is required, yet more nutrients reach the blood and cells.

One of the easiest proteins to assimilate is chlorophyl. The sprouting process, under the action of light, creates it. Chlorophyl has been shown in many instances to be effective in overcoming protein-deficiency anemia (39).

Since the general pattern of distribution of essential amino acids in legume and cereal protein in dissimilar, when needed, they are capable of supplementing each other with the result that legume-cereal mixtures contain protein of increased nutritive value. Dr. S. Kuppuswammy of the Indian Council of Medical Research in his review (10) of protein in food, brings this out factually. As an example, it has been proven that chick peas and wheat protein supplement each other, giving you a complete protein. In the same study, it has been shown that the growth promoting value and the digestibility of chick peas is increased with germination.

There is a great deal of controversy over heat processing of legumes to increase protein digestibility. According (10) to S. Kuppuswammy: "There are a number of reports in the literature to the effect that the nutritive value of pea protein is impaired as the result of heat-processing. Controversy exists also regarding the effect of heat-processing on the biological value of protein present in numerous other legumes, such as chick peas, lentils, mung beans . . . Many legumes contain trypsin (a pancreatic enzyme which releases lysine and arginine from protein structure) inhibitor which in most cases is heat-liable, but no correlation has been observed between the effect of autoclaving (steam heating) on the nutritive value of protein and the presence or absence of trypsin inhibitor in the raw legume. Soy bean, which is so commonly used as a source of protein, was found to improve the digestibility and biological value after heating."

The trypsin controversy was resolved recently by Kakade and Evans (146) and Hegazi (147). Their studies showed clearly that germination eliminates the inhibitor.

The destructiveness of heat on protein is well documented in the following experiments. Evans and Butts (40) showed that under typical cooking conditions, the lysine loss was 50% by chemical analysis or 84% loss by enzymatic analysis. E.M. Olsen (41) heat treated wheat germ. Because of chemical changes, the absorption ability of amino acids is dramatically altered. The overall effect of nitrogen absorption was reduced to as low as 63%. On specific amino acids, there was a reduction of lysine absorption to 42% and 54, 56 and 58 percent for isoleucine, valine, and leucine respectively.

We have seen from previous studies that sprouting increases the quality of protein, likewise it removes the inhibitor factors, hence it is the preferred method of treating seeds.

Thus we see it would be preferable to eat raw protein. We overcome the problem of the inhibitors by noting that they are not only heat sensitive, but also water soluble. During sprouting they are washed away. Considering that sprouted legumes—soybeans, mung beans, lentils and alfalfa—are an important staple for many earthlings, and considering the good health of those who eat little food and who eat their sprouts raw, one need not worry about inhibitors.

SPROUT A COMPLETE PROTEIN

There are two ways to establish whether a food item supplies a complete protein. First through biological studies using animals (or by observing cultural diet patterns of humans) who eat a controlled diet. If adequate protein is present, then the researchers expect a normal growth rate, absence of classical protein deficiency diseases, longevity pattern of that species and healthy reproduction for at least several generations. Second, through chemical analysis.

By the first method, Dr. Francis Pottenger, Jr. had found *"sprouted grain to be complete protein in an animal test, completely servicing the reproduction program through generations (p. 40) . . . he had found sprouted legumes and grains to contribute enough first quality protein to be classed as complete (26, p. 295)."* Likewise, Dr. C.F. Schnabel showed grass is adequate in providing all needed nutrients, including protein, in animal experiments (115).

To establish by the second method one has to take the indirect approach because of lack of nutritional data on sprouts.

From the study of germination process, Drs. Mayer and Poljakoff-Mayber (Germination of Seed, Pergamon Press, 1963) of the Botany Dept., Hebrew University, Jerusalem, observed: *"Nitrogen (protein) appears to be very carefully conserved. In place of the protein broken down there appears free amino acids and amides."* That is, in germination, the amino acids are freed (not destroyed) from their protein structure. Hence, if a seed contains a complete protein then the sprout (of lower density due to the dilluting effect of water) can be anticipated to contain all the amino acids that were in the original seed protein. From the following table (Amino Acid Content of Food, Orr and Watt, Wash., D.C.) we see that the listed seeds

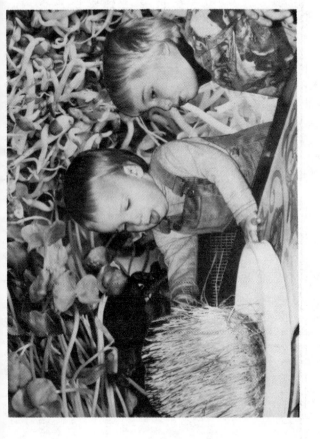

Sprouts Are Coming.

Chick peas + wheat = Complete protein   Seeds + Sprouts are (separately) Complete Protein

TABLE 3

	chick peas	soy sprout	buck wheat	buck sprout	human milk av.	max.	sun flower	sunflower sprout
tryptophan	0.170		.17	.03	.058	.103	0.343	.06
threonine	0.739	0.017	.46	.09	.257	.284	0.911	.15
isoleusine	1.195	0.159	.44	.09	.240	.344	1.276	.21
leucine	1.538	0.225	.68	.15	.475	.567	1.736	.30
lysine	1.434	0.265	.69	.16	.353	.413	0.868	.12
methionine	0.276	0.211	.21	.04	.051	.128	0.443	.07
phenylalanine	1.012	0.045	.44	.09	.142	.272	1.220	.20
valine	1.025	0.186	.61	.12	.283	.391	1.354	.21
argine	1.551	.225	.93	.19	.172	.253	2.370	.30
histidine	0.559	.133	.26	.05	.061	.138	0.586	.09
total protein	28%	6%	12%	2%	.8%	1.4%	23%	4%

	lentil	soy	mung	sesame	wheat	date	egg	meat
tryptophan	0.216	0.526	0.180	.33	0.173	.06	.211	0.220
threonine	0.896	1.504	0.765	.71	0.403	.06	.637	0.830
isoleusine	1.316	2.054	1.351	.95	0.607	.07	.850	0.984
leucine	1.760	2.946	2.202	1.7	0.939	.08	1.126	1.540
lysine	1.528	2.414	1.667	.58	0.384	.07	.819	1.642
methionine	0.180	0.513	0.265	.64	0.214	.03	.401	0.466
phenylalanine	1.104	1.889	1.167	1.5	0.691	.06	.739	0.773
valine	1.360	2.005	1.440	.89	0.648	.09	.950	1.044
argine	1.908	2.763	1.370	1.9	0.670	.05	.840	1.212
histidine	0.548	0.911	0.543	.44	0.286	.05	.307	0.653
total protein	25%	35%	24.4%	19%	14%	2.2%	13%	19%

Sunflower and Buckwheat sprout values are my own approximation.

contain a complete protein. Hence the sprouts of the seeds are also complete proteins.

The table values are for raw produce. Pasteurized dairy produce, eggs and meat do not have the amino acids listed in the table when they are served in the cooked form. Without any considerations, if one is to search for a food item that would supply a complete protein, one would choose raw sprouted seeds.

MY MINERAL MINE

It has been observed that people who drink mineral water are healthier than those who drink soft water. It is also rumored that Romans who drank water in which rusty swords were soaked cured their anemia, also, clay taken internally heals broken bones through its silica.

It might be true that the hard mineral water drinker is healthier than the soft water drinker. However, the most dramatic effect of maintaining health, as well as regeneration is produced by drinking organic minerals in the form of fresh juices. The heavy inorganic mineral water might be producing a temporary improvement in some aspect of health, but the overall affect is a build up of inorganic minerals which leads to the arthritic condition of old age.

Some of the reasons why the inorganic minerals seem to be useful toward maintenance of health are as follow:

(1). The inorganic minerals might help to neutralize other inorganic toxic minerals, as well as toxic waste within the system.

(2). Alkaline inorganic minerals can osmotically draw out toxins from the system into the intestinal tract, as well as produce a mild laxative effect.

(3). The drinking of water containing the iron of swords might have helped to overcome anemia for reasons 1 or 2; or merely by drinking lots of water whether the swords were soaked in it or not, could reduce and flush out toxemia, leading to recovery.

(4). It is very hard to pin point exactly the reasons for a recovery and whether the inorganic iron played a role in the healing. As an example, doctors used crude chlorophyll in the successful treatment of many forms of anemia, yet they were not able to determine the exact factor for regeneration of the hemoglobin level, which could have been due to: The use of dietary chlorophyll to build the hemoglobin; or, the chlorophyll acted as a stimulant—a vibratory pattern—for the building of more hemoglobin from other material.

ORGANIC MINERAL LOSS

The ability of body to utilize inorganic minerals is very limited. Individuals who expect ferrous sulfate pill to supply the minimal daily requirements of the bloodstream are cheated. In studies done, scientists found that absorption of inorganic iron into the bloodstream was as low as 3.8% of the dose taken.

Some of the reasons for poor iron transport can be found in the stomach where the iron salt is ionized. The positively charged iron is attracted to the negatively charged intestine, where it sticks to it, irritating the lining. Body may generate excess fluid to flush out the irritation. Minerals are lost in this manner.

Another reason for the unavailability of iron in the bloodstream is due to the formation of insoluble compounds with other food elements, such as phosphates (phytic acid). The acid combines well with calcium, iron, zinc and other minerals, which reduce significantly their absorption into the bloodstream. Similarly, oxalic acid of spinach can reduce significantly the availability of calcium.

Phytin is very frequently present in many seeds and may constitute up to 80% of the phosphorous content of the seed (3). The absolute amount of phytin varies in species and families. For example, wheat phytin contains 12% calcium and 1.5% magnesium, while oat phytin is 8.3% calcium and 15% magnesium (150).

Hence, eating a diet rich in seed, besides the high protein complications, can result in a tremendous loss of important minerals, in spite of the fact that seeds are rich sources of such minerals. However, the mineral losses because of the high phytin concentration become insignificant if one sprouts the seeds.

Drs. Mayer and Poljakoff-Mayber (3) of Hebrew University state that most of phytin disappears in the seeds studied:

> *"Some of the phosphorous containing compounds occurring in cotton seed and the changes in them during germination are shown in the following table . . . the large amount of phytin present may be regarded as a store of inorganic phosphate which is liberated as germination proceeds . . . by enzyme phytase . . . In oats, phytase activity in the entire seeds seems to*

TABLE:

CHANGES IN PHYTIN CONTENT OF COTTON SEED MG PHOSPHOROUS PER GRAM DRY WEIGHT

days of germination	0	1	4	6
	8.61	8.94	4.00	1.97

(Plant Phys. 34,476,1959)

develop rather slowly and the total phytin content decreases to about a half in the course of a week. In wheat, on the other hand, most of the phytin has disappeared after a similar period."

Likewise, the doctors (3) found the increase of desirable forms of phosphorous compounds:

"Early work on phospholipids, and especially lecithin, in a number of seeds tends to support an increase in phospholipids during germination. This was usually the case for seeds germinated in light."

Thus we see that sprouting increases the amount of lecithin, and by reducing phytin, sprouting increases the availability to the blood of the alkalizing minerals. The availability of minerals can be further increased by the following process.

CHELATED MINERALS

The binding of an inorganic mineral to an organic molecule, such as an amino acid, is the process known as chelation. This builds a fence around the mineral protecting it from chemical reaction within the intestinal tract. This increases absorption and utilization within the body.

All natures laboratories use chelation. Only recently it has been applied in the health food industry. Among the chelated compounds in nature are hemoglobin of the blood, chlorophyll in plants and most enzymes in live food.

Basically, as already mentioned, many important dietary minerals can be lost by either forming compounds which the body cannot utilize or by having the minerals stick to the intestinal tract due to electrical polarity, which lead to irritation and flushing out as waste of the minerals.

However, when the minerals enter the body in a chelated form, i.e. bound to an amino structure, they are relatively stable which prevents the minerals from forming new compounds with other nutrients and from sticking to the intestinal lining.

Dr. Ashmead, at the International College of Applied Nutrition meeting in Los Angeles in April, 1974, told of the chelation process in the body, where the bond had to be just right to prevent problems of mineral availability.

A weak bond such as iron citrate leads to release of iron in stomach where it can interact with other nutrients, such as phytic acid, to form iron phosphate, which cannot be utilized by the body. A strong bond, such as in EDTA, never releases the mineral for use by the body.

In the human system, the liver, a major chelating agent, takes minerals from the bloodstream and forms chelates. Dr. Ashmead said there are no free metal ions, except those that are in the process of becoming chelates. When minerals in our diet are in chelated form their availability to the bloodstream is increased many times. In chelated form, magnesium is absorbed about 2.5 times as great as in sulfate form; copper 5.8 times as great than the carbonate form; iron 3 times more than the sulfate form (Prevention, Nov., 1974).

Sprouted seeds are the best sources of natural chelates. In the germination process, the complex proteins of seeds are broken down into amino acids. The acids are hooked up to a mineral and a vitamin, forming a natural chelate, called an enzyme. From the previous discussion, as well as the following table, we see that seeds when sprouted are the highest natural source of enzymes, hence of chelated minerals.

TABLE:

GERMINATION OF PEANUT

Enzyme activity expressed in umoles glycomate

time days	length of sprout tail (mm)	Enzyme Activity	
		isocitritase	malate synthetase
0	0	—	—
1	0	0	0
2	2	7.9	10.2
3	16	20.4	24.6
4	35	30.0	50.2
5	55	42.3	69.4

(J. Biol. Chem. 235, 563, 1960)

THE SPROUT CONSPIRACY

The sproutarian menu is being challenged as a valuable source of nutrients by a few of today's journals. They are stacked with 'convincing evidence' that a hamburger might be a more sensible choice for the next meal. Here are some representative articles:

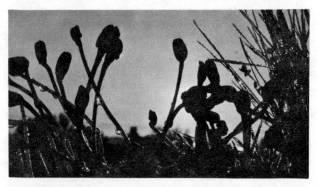

Rising Sun, wheatgrass and sunflower greens.

The following is a letter received by a friend from the Quaker Oats Company, nutritional research department:

January 15, 1976

Mr. Phillip D. Bird
400 East First Street
Northfield, Minnesota 55057

Dear Mr. Bird:

Jack Gould has requested that I answer your letter of January 10, 1976.

We have done some work on sprouting oats but unfortunately we only worked with the grain after it was sprouted for a short time in the absence of light.

No feeding trials have been made by Quaker with either the sprouts or germinated seed as our objective was not oriented toward the nutritional aspects of this process.

Some studies of the nutritional quality of sprouted grains for both ruminant and monogastric animals have been made in Europe. Florentin and Florentin,

Bull, Acad. vet. France vol. 34 page 93, 1966 found the following composition for oat sprouts germinated for three days and grown hydroponically for 5 days; protein 1.62%, non-protein nitrogen 3.35%, fat 1.95%, starch 7.89%, sugars 6.63%, cellulose 2.10%, crude fiber 2.96%, ash 1.67%, water by difference 71.83%.

Oat forage at early dough stage maturity was found to have: protein 9.23%, crude fiber 30.44%, nitrogen free extract 49.33%, fat 3.56% and ash 44%. These figures were taken from "Forages, the Science of land Agriculture". H.D. Hughes et al Ed's, Iowa State College Press, Ames, Iowa, p. 395.

There have been many claims made about the increase in nutritional value of germinated grains. However, I failed to find a scientifically sound reference in Chemical Abstracts from 1937 to 1971 and none in Nutrition Abstracts 1955 to 1971. It would be reasonable to assume that some increase would occur in provitamin A in the sprouts but B^{12} and D would still be deficient in a diet that was based on such materials.

From a nutritional standpoint using sprouts rather than the grain is a poor trade. The grain is a low moisture, high energy and fair to excellent source of protein wrapped in a stable package. The sprouts are high moisture, low energy, poor sources of protein. They also are quite high in fiber and ash content which may cause difficulty in the monogastric animal. As a ready year round source of salad greens and to enable variety in the diet they are excellent but as a serious contender for a part in human diets they would require more sophisticated technology than the householder would have available. It is the same situation as with leaf protein where in theory it could solve the world need for protein but the technology to utilize it is some distance in the future.

As far as the seeds are concerned the longer the period of germination the less nutritional value could be recovered. The seed is a source of nutrients for the seedling and a large portion of protein, carbohydrate and fat are consumed before photosynthesis becomes adequate to maintain the seedling.

I hope that the above does not sound as if Quaker is not interested in the huge task of adequately feeding our burgeoning population. We all realize the enormity of the problem and have been active in the area of improving both nutritional and agronomic qualities of corn and oats as well as formulation of less expensive but nutritive foods.

If we can be of further service please feel free to ask.

Sincerely yours,
George C. Potter, Ph.D.
Manager Lipid Research

FEDS DOUBT SPROUT TOUT

Health-food restaurant owners are queasy these days, because of spreading awareness of a book published by the U.S. Department of Agriculture. In it are facts that threaten to turn their world topsy-turvy. The facts: Bean sprouts, despite their health-food reputation, are only moderately nutritious. On the whole they have less to offer than an equal weigh of boiled lima beans.

Composition of Foods, the book which gives chemical analyses of nearly 2500 foodstuffs, reports on the two commonest sprouts: sprouted mung beans, the familiar "chop suey" sprouts, and sprouted soybeans. Mung sprouts are greatly inferior to soy sprouts, as are more exotic sprouts (not listed in the book) such as alfalfa. This is because most of the nutrition found in a sprout is present in the unsprouted seed, and the soybean is the most nutritious of seeds to begin with.

Weight for weight, the data show, soy sprouts

have about the same amount of calcium as lima beans: about 80% as much vitamin C and protein; about half as much food energy, phosphorus and iron; and less than a third as much vitamin A. They surpass limas only in two B vitamins, having 25% more thiamine and twice as much riboflavin; about as much, in other words, as enriched white bread. Soy sprouts have only half the niacin of lima beans.

As sprout enthusiasts point out, sprouting is a form of agriculture that requires neither soil nor sunlight. This is the reason, in fact, for sprouts' mediocre showing—they have never taken minerals from soil or photosynthesized food energy like a green plant. Except in vitamin A and C content, soy sprouts are weight for weight far less nutritious than unsprouted soybeans.

The content of vitamins A and C does increase with sprouting, but the end product is a bulky way to obtain vitamins. You would have to eat about four cups of soy sprouts to get the amount of vitamin A found in half a good-sized tomato. As for vitamin C, soy sprouts have less of it than an equal weight of french-fried potatoes.

(Rolling Stone, No. 203, 1976)

It is of virtue to compare different researchers regarding the nutritional effect of germination upon seeds. It seems on the surface that the U.S. Department of Agriculture, via its publication "Composition of Foods" (9), is trying to discourage sprouting. There seems to be a loss of nutrients. The vitamin C was the only one recorded to increase in value.

TABLE 4

Dry	Thiamin		Riboflavin		Niacin	
Source	(17)	(9)	(17)	(9)	(17)	(9)
Dry Soybean	.88	.38	.12	.21	3.0	3.6
4 day old			.26		5.1	
5 day old	1.03		1.0		7.0	
germinated	1.03	.13	1.0	.10	7.0	.7

(17) Burkholder and McVeigh, Yale University
(9) Composition of Foods, Department of Agriculture

The reason for the difference, is that one is calculated on a dry base (17) while the other on a wet base (9). The former enables you to see that there has been an increase in vitamin content. The latter figure is smaller because the moisture content in the beans increased at a rate much faster than the vitamin content. Vitamin content per seed increased because of germination.

The 'junk eaters' have very little intake of these live nutrients. The following comparative values are listed by the Department of Agriculture (9):

TABLE 5

Quick cooking wheat and
    barley cereal (no. 2453)........01 mg/100 gr. of vit. B2
Flour, enriched all purpose........05 mg/100 gr. of vit. B2
White Bread (no. 465)..............08 mg/100 gr. of vit. B2
Wheat (27)..............................13 mg/100 gr. of vit. B2
Wheat sprout (27).....................54 mg/100 gr. of vit. B2

Vitamin value increase is tremendous during sprouting. In Nutrition Review (4) the author speaks on vitamin B-complex: "Greater than can be accounted for by loss of dried matter. Hence, you are getting free vitamins." In other reviews (5, 6) the rapid synthesis of provitamins A and vitamin C in germinating seed has been clearly demonstrated by many investigators in recent years.

Total protein content per mung bean seed rose on the average from 25% in the dry seed to 37% in the dried sprout. A similar increase was observed in the sprouted soybean (122). Thus there was a total 12% protein increase per seed due to the sprouting process.

Dr. Burkholder of Yale in Science (27) states: "Germinated peas and buckwheat showed gains in pyridoxine and folic acid ranging from 3 to 10 fold and smaller increases in pantothenic acid . . . The data obtained thus far strongly supports that view that many seeds gain in vitamin content during germination. The common use of sprouted seed of Oriental people in diet rest on sound nutritional content of such material."

VITAMINS IN NATURE

Untampered natural food has the power to build blood, tissue, nerves, bone and maintain life. When food is fragmented, reduced to individual component parts, and then reproduced synthetically, these parts are incomplete and will have missing many valuable factors. As an example, an essential vitamin B12, which has been only recently identified, was missing in the synthetic supplements as well as cooked diet, however, it had been supplied to the users of natural vitamins.

Vitamins in their natural state are those found in

natural foods and are accompanied by their coexisting enzymes, minerals, amino acids and other naturally occurring synergists (co-workers). Although popularly not accepted as fact, there are many researchers (132, 133, 134) who believe that natural vitamin complexes as existing in natural foods contain valuable food components not found in any synthetic vitamins.

Dr. Pottenger (135) in a 10 year experiment demonstrated that processed foods lead to degenerative diseases. Total breakdown in reproductive capacity by third generation. Animals fed raw, natural food lived generation after generation in health.

VITAMIN INCREASE DURING SPROUTING

Vitamin value increase is tremendous during sprouting. In Nutrition Review (4) the author speaks on vitamin B-complex: "The changes in the vitamin content, however, are much greater than can be accounted for by loss of dried matter. Hence, you are getting free vitamins." In other reviews (5, 6) the rapid synthesis of provitamins A and vitamin C in germinating seed has been clearly demonstrated by many investigators in recent years.

Dr. Burkholder of Yale in Science (27) states: "Germinated peas and buckwheat showed gains in pyridoxine and folic acid ranging from 3 to 10 fold and smaller increases in pantothenic acid . . . The data obtained thus far strongly supports the view that many seeds gain in vitamin content during germination. The common use of sprouted seed of Oriental people in diet rest on sound nutritional content of such material."

Studies in India showed that the eight legumes and two grains studied all had a significant increase in carotene, vitamin A Precursor (20). By sprouting the

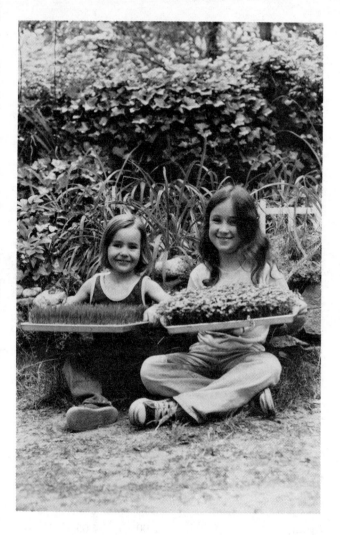

Children of Light —wheatgrass and buckwheat.

Photo by Mary Ann Sacchetti

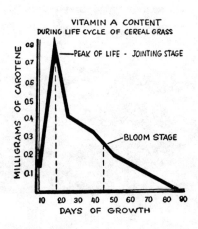

VITAMIN A CONTENT
DURING LIFE CYCLE OF CEREAL GRASS

PEAK OF LIFE - JOINTING STAGE

BLOOM STAGE

MILLIGRAMS OF CAROTENE

DAYS OF GROWTH

wheat for several days you can expect at least double the carotene content. If the sprout is allowed to mature on soil, the wheat cereal grass part content is 75,000 I.U. carotene per pound, more than twice the amount found in carrots (25). The Biblical expression, "and their eyes failed because there was no grass to eat," seems to be well founded.

TABLE 6
CAROTENE CONTENT OF PULSES AND
CEREAL (21) MG/100G

Name	Days of Germination			
	0	2	4	7
Lentil	1.60	2.00	4.05	—
Chick Pea	2.54	3.54	4.30	—
Mung bean	2.9	4.07	4.25	—
Rice	.35	.75	2.15	3.95
Wheat	.45	.70	2.25	4.65

Other studies of Asiatic origin reported by Wai et al showed (32) Bansey soybeans grown in the dark at 28 deg. C doubled the carotene content in 48 hours, increased 2.8 times in 54 hours and 3.4 times in 72 hours. Thiamin showed a slight gain in 24 hours. Riboflavin increased 100% after 54 hours. Nicotinic acid doubled in 72 hours (37).

Dr. C.W. Bailey of the University of Minnesota, disclosed that vitamin C value during the early sprouting period of wheat increased by 600% (26).

An indepth study (27) by Dr. Burkholder of Yale University brings out why "you can take the Orient out of Asia, but not the sprouties out of the Orient."

TABLE 7
VITAMINS IN DRY SEEDS AND IN GERMINATED SEEDS
RESULTS EXPRESSED AS MICROGRAMS PER GRAM OF
DRY MATTER

Kind of Seed	Treatment	Riboflavin
Wheat	Dry	1.0
	Soaked	1.4
	4 Days old	2.4
Corn	Dry	1.5
	Soaked	0.5
	4 Days old	2.0
Soy bean	Dry	1.8
	Soaked	1.4
	4 Days Old	3.6
Mung bean	Dry	1.2
	Soaked	1.2
	4 Days old	2.6
	5 Days old	10.0

TABLE 8

VITAMIN CONTENT (MICROGRAMS PER GRAM) OF DRY SEEDS AND OF SEEDS GERMINATED FOR 5 DAYS IN SAND CULTURES

Kind of Seed	Riboflavin		Niacin		Thiamine		Biotin	
	Dry	Germin.	Dry	Germin.	Dry	Germin.	Dry	Germin.
Barley	1.3	8.3	72	129	.....	7.9	0.4	1.2
Corn	1.2	3.0	17	40	6.2	5.5	0.3	0.7
Oats	0.6	12.4	11	48	10.0	11.5	1.2	1.8
Soy bean	2.0	9.1	27	49	10.7	9.6	1.1	3.5
Lima (large)	1.0	2.0	15	29	6.7	5.0	0.1	0.1
Lima (small)	0.9	4.0	11	41	4.5	6.2	0.1	0.4
Green eye pea	1.8	9.7	20	60	11.0	12.0	0.4	1.1
Mung bean	1.2	10.0	26	70	8.8	10.3	0.2	1.0
Pea	0.7	7.3	31	32	7.2	9.2	.....	0.5

TABLE 9
(Values Given in Microgram Per Gram of Dry Matter.)

	Wheat		Oat		Barley		Corn	
	Dor-mant	Sprout	Dor-mant	Sprout	Dor-mant	Sprout	Dor-mant	Sprout
Dry matter mg. per seed	28.5	21.4	19.3	14.8	35.6	30.2	31.5	271.
Riboflavin	1.3	5.4	.8	11.6	.9	7.2	1.1	4.3
Nicotinic Acid	62.0	103.0	7.5	44.	67.5	115.	9.5	39.5
Biotin	.17	.36	.9	1.4	.31	.91	.21	.54
Panthonthenic Acid	7.6	12.6	7.6	21.9	5.4	10.	4.2	7.7
Pyridoxine	2.6	4.6	.3	1.8	.2	.5	.7	.8
Folic Acid	28.0	106.0	22.	143.	14.5	50.	10.	45.
Inositol	1460.	2100.	630.	1290.	1240.	1370.	800.	1640.
Thiamin	7.	9.	11.3	12.2	6.8	9.	5.5	5.5

Sprouts continue to be an important staple of the American Chinese and Japanese. The following tables 7, 8 and 9 (17, 27) is from his study on the vitamin B complex in grains and legumes.

We might note from table 8 in wheat, vitamin B2 increased 400 percent, vitamin B1 by 29 percent. In oat, vitamin B2 increase was 1450% as the result of germination. You are getting a tremendous amount of vitamins at little expense of time and money.

> Dr. Burkholder concluded, "If the food value of germinated seeds is to be judged by their content of vitamins and readily available amino acids, then it appears that the common use of sprouts in the diets of Oriental peoples rests on a sound nutritional basis and should be introduced on a wide scale among Occidentals."

VITAMIN B-12 SOURCES

Many nutritionists base their criticism of vegetarianism on the dietary absence of the anti-pernicious vitamin B-12. They overlook the fact that this vitamin is heat sensitive and over 85% (137) of its effectiveness can be lost under normal cooking conditions. Since no one eats raw meat, the nutritionist cannot make claim to animal protein as being a source of this vitamin. Then, the question has to be raised why are we not having a wide spread planetary epidemic of pernicious anemia?

At a recent conference on vitamin B-12, it was revealed that the ultimate source of all vitamin B-12 is certain bacteria (136). It seems that vitamin B-12 needs of human and animal is adequately supplied by the intestinal tract bacteria.

The main courses of development of vitamin B-12 deficiency are as following:

(1) a thick coating of mucus and slime along the intestinal tract, which reduces permability to all vitamins.

(2) Putrefactive bacteria predominate due to such factors as overeating, bad mixtures of food, high protein diet, excess sugar, smog, enzyme deficiency, insecticides.

The most pronounced symptom of vitamin B-12 deficiency is extreme sensitivity to heat and cold—normal tap water feels like ice, with pins and needle pain on skin. I have had these symptoms. I have also observed it in six other individuals, all vegetarians.

The common cause was a combination of factors of dietary origin. The condition was quickly corrected in 3 to 10 days, depending on the individual, by following good food combination, eating only when hungry, eliminating all sweets, cutting down on protein, increasing the greens and sprouts in ones diet. The putrefactive bacteria, with associated gas, was replaced by friendly bacteria which are noted for the manufacture of the B-complex vitamins, including the B-12.

The experience at Hippocrates Health Institute (48) as well as the clinic studies in medical journals (79), summerized in my other (49) text, point to the ability of successfully treating anemia with chlorophyl rich juice. The chlorophyl treatment (138) also gives successful results with pernicious anemia.

The sproutarians are further guaranteed more than a full quanta of vitamin B-12 from sprouts. Daily serving of several cups of sprouts will supply more than the known daily requirements (24) of this vitamin.

However, the best source of vitamin B-12 is the intestinal tract bacteria. They will be the major source of this nutrient as long as one follows good eating habits (49) which discourage the growth of the putrefactive intestinal bacteria.

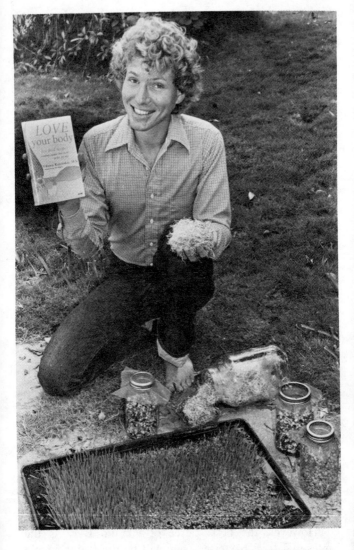

Joshua Lane, teaching how to meet the RDDR on sprouts.

TABLE 10
VITAMIN B-12 CONTENT, MG/G

Name	Days of Germination		
	0	2	4
Mung bean	.61	.81	1.53
Lentil	.43	.42	2.37
Chick Pea	.35	1.90	1.22
Green Pea	.36	1.27	2.36

MEETING THE RECOMMENDED
DAILY DIETARY REQUIREMENTS

In examining the tables of minimal dietary requirements (136) we see a range of values for each nutrient depending on the age of the individual.

I choose the dietary need values for a healthy detoxified grown up as the ones that the nutritionist suggest for babies.

Why? Because a baby still has a relatively uncongested intestinal tract with a high nutrient permeability. More nutrients can be trasported to the blood and cells when the tract is not coated with mucus and slime, or is hardened and scared due to the dietary abuses. A detoxified individual on a mucus lean diet will have even a cleaner intestinal tract than the typical polluted bloodstream baby. Such an individual has an even lower dietary needs than recommended for a baby.

The protein daily requirement is 32 grams (136). The healthy Hunzas, strong Georgians and the long lived Equartorians of Vilcabamba based on a 1973 study (143) are starving themselves to a long, joyous full life on a dietary daily intake of 35 grams protein,

1200 calories and 12 grams of fat, all from natural foods. They are a good example of semi detoxified individuals, who do very well through undernourishment in the complex nutrients—fats, protein and starch —and over nourish in vitamins, minerals and enzymes from natures food.

The following suggestions for meeting the RDDA requirements are based on referenced material and tables found in the text.

TABLE 11
RECOMMENDED DAILY DIETARY ALLOWANCES (136)

| | Toxic Human** | | Extrapolations by Viktoras based on health* |
	Max. table value		
Vitamin A	5.000 I.U.	2.500 I.U.	2.500 I.U.
Thiamine	1.4 mg	.6 mg.	.6 mg.
Riboflavin	2.0 mg.	.6 mg.	.6 mg.
Niacin	22 mg.	7 mg.	7 mg.
Ascorbic Acid	80 mg.	40 mg.	40 mg.
Calcium	1.4 g.	.8 mg.	.8 mg.
Iron	15 mg.	10 mg.	10 mg.
Protein	85 g.	32 g.	32 g.
Calories	2.900	1.600	1.600

*mucuslean organic diet, non polluted environment

**Much higher values are desirable when an individual leads a high stress life of a city, especially on a mucus, processed non-organic diet. The subject is well covered by authors like Adele Davis, Carlton Fredericks, Paavo Airola, as well as the many articles found in Prevention Magazine. The basis for the RDDA is discussed by Max Huberman (Let's Live, March 1976, p. 50). Best supplement for city survival is a daily dose of at least 8 oz. of juice from weeds, sprouts, grass, greens.

Vitamin A requirements (2500 I.U.) can be met by eating daily any of the following foods: ½ pound papaya, 1/5 pound of mango. The juice from ⅛ pound spinach, 1/10 pound of carrots or 1/15 pound of wheatgrass or dandelion will likewise supply an adequate amount of vitamin A.

Thiamine (.6 mg) can be met from: 3 oz. unhulled sesame, 1.5 oz. sunflower, ½ oz. mung bean or wheat sprout.

Riboflavin (.6 mg) requirements can be supplied by 9 oz. dandelion, 10 oz. avocado, 9 oz. unhulled sesame, ½ oz, wheatsprout, ¼ oz. mung bean sprout.

Vitamin C (40 mg) can be supplied from 3 oz. mung bean or soy sprout, 1 oz. sweet red pepper, 5 oz. papaya, 5 oz. spinach, 6 oz. orange juice.

The calcium requirements of .8 grams can be supplied by 3 oz. unhulled sesame seed, 12 oz. parsley or dandelion greens.

The RDDA figure for calcium (as well as for other nutrients) are based on an acid producing diet of meat, starch and fat. Lots of calcium is required to neutralize this acid condition. On a vegetarian diet, by consuming fresh greens sprouts and alkaline fruit, the individual will not be acidifying the body and the calcium requirements will be met by even a small quantity of food.

Iron needs can be supplied by 3 oz. sesame, ⅓ oz. dulse or kelp, 10 oz. spinach, 5 oz. sunflower seed. These requirements are also excessive (49) due to the high cellular death on an acid producing diet.

Protein (32 grams) needs can be met with 4 oz. of sesame, 1.5 pounds of mung bean sprout. These values are also far too extreme.

To discover a better approximation of the true dietary needs for a health detoxified individual one should examine the composition of mother's breast milk. This fluid supplies the protein needs of a baby during the period of most rapid growth and development. It has on the average 1 gram of protein per 100 grams of fluid. A baby drinks approximately one quart of milk in a 24 hour period. This would supply about 10 grams of protein. Such quantity can come from 8 oz. of mung sprouts of 1.5 oz. sesame or 2 oz. wheat sprout, or 5 pounds papaya or 4 pounds mango.

ALFALFA

Alfalfa, though the smallest of seed in the legume family, turns out to be the favorite. Nutritionally it should be superior to all other sprouts for it is very selective and has roots that extend up to 100 feet into the earth to seek out minerals and other nutrients. Americans are willing to pay up to $4.00 per pound to enjoy alfalfa sprouts in their salads.

Alfalfa (47) is one of the most complete and nutritionally rich of all foods tested. In addition to a fabulously high potency of vitamins as well as minerals, it is high in protein and contains every essential amino acid, its anti-toxin or detoxification properties surpass those of every food tested: liver, brewer's yeast, and wheat germ. It has been found to provide resistance to disease and seems to help these ailments which end in "itis" such as arthritis. It also helps to prevent exhaustion and provides an excellent calcium-phosphorus ratio (2:1).

The well documented book (33) Nature's Healing Grasses by Dr. H.E. Kirschner, M.D. says that the researcher Frank Bower showed green alfalfa to contain eight essential enzymes which are necessary for good digestion.

TABLE 12
Analysis of Dehydrated Alfalfa Greens
per 100 Grams

Vitamins		Minerals	
A	up to 44,000 i.u.	Phosphorous	250 mg.
D	1,040 i.u.	Calcium	1,750 mg.
E	50 i.u.	Potassium	2,000 mg.
K	15 i.u.	Sodium	150 mg.
U	unknown	Chlorine	280 mg.
C	176 mg.	Sulfur	290 mg.
B-1	0.8 mg.	Magnesium	310 mg.
B-2	1.8 mg.	Copper	2 mg.
B-6	1.0 mg.	Manganese	5 mg.
B-12	0.3 mcg.	Iron	35 mg.
Niacin	5 mg.	Cobalt	2.4 mg.
Panthothenic Acid	3.3 mg.	Boron	4.7 mg.
Inositol	210 mg.	Molybdenum	2.6 ppm
Biotin	033 mg.		
Folic Acid	0.8 mg.	Trace Minerals	
		Nickel	
Other Content		Strontium	
Fiber	25%	Lead	
Protein	20%	Paladium	
Fat Solubles	3%		
i.u. = international units		mg. = milligram	
ppm = parts per million		mcg. = microgram	

Alfalfa seed (10) Indian variety Ranger (Medicago Sativa) can have a protein content as high as 39.8 percent and contains all the essential amino acids: Isoleucine (3.7%), Leucine (7.4%), Lysine (4.2%), Methionine (1.3%), Tryptophone (.7%), Threonine Phenylalaine (4.2%), Valine (4.4%).

If you grow on soil, protein content (34) of the aerial part when dried can vary from 16.4 to 30.5 percent depending upon fertilizer and environmental factors.

The percentage of protein in sprouts is inversely related to the increase in weight. The alfalfa sprout increases approximately seven fold in weight over the seed, hence we would expect the protein content of alfalfa sprouts to be between 2 and 5 percent.

A book of tables on metabolism (25) reports that undried alfalfa leaves can be as high as 5.2 percent protein. However, in the sprouted seed the value will be much lower. Carotene level is about the same as found in carrot. Because of its long roots the leaves contain a wide range of minerals (25): calcium, iron, magnesium, potassium, phosphorus, sodium, sulphur, cobalt, and zinc.

Experiments (35) have been done by Binger, Thompson and Kohler, chemists of the Western Utilization Development Division to relate the productivity of alfalfa to the quality of the soil. The seeds were sorted on a 15.5, 20.6 and 24.8 percent protein level and the corresponding vitamin values were determined. Here are the results:

TYPICAL ANALYSIS OF DEHYDRATED UNJOINTED GRASS AND OF ALFALFA

	Unjointed Cereal Grass	Alfalfa		Unjointed Cereal Grass	Alfalfa
Solid	95%	95%	Folic Acid	5	4
Protein	20%	17%	Folinic Acid mg./lb.	*(2)	***?
Ether extractives	8%	6%	Thiamine mg/lb.	5	3
Mineral (ash)	12%	12%	Pyridoxine mg/lb.	6	6
Fiber	17%	25%	Ascorbic acid mg/lb.	1600	700
Vitamin A (carotene)			Choline mg/lb.	470	500
IU/lb.	300,000	150,000	Inositol mg/lb.	300	950
Vitamin K mg/lb.	70	35	Betaine mg/lb.	***?	2000
Vitamin E mg/lb.	150	110	Vitamin B12 mcg./lb. ...	20	20
Riboflavin	11	7	Biotin mcg./lb.	500	150
Niacin mg/lb.	35	18	Thioctic acid mcg./lb.	1100	**275
Pantothenic mg/lb.	11	16			

*This figure does not represent the dehydrated product but is a calculated figure based on an analysis of juice. Conventional dehydration destroys most of this factor.
**Leaf meal   ***No data available

TABLE 13
DEHYDRATED ALFALFA MEAL PROTEIN LEVEL

Vitamin	15.5% mg/100g	20.6% mg/100g	24.8% mg/100g
FAT SOLUBE			
B-Carotene	9.6	20.3	23.2
Xanthophylls	19.3	48.3	50.7
Total Tocopherol (vit. E)	15.8	19.1	20.1
Vitamin K	1.61	2.16	1.84
WATER SOLUBE			
Riboflavin	.31	1.59	.60
Thiamin	2.89	5.3	4.86
Panthothenic Acid	3.91	5.13	5.44
Niacin	.57	.504	.91
Pyridoxine	.57	.90	3.13
Inositol	.58	2.16	3.7
Folic Acid	.18	.36	1.69
Choline	98.	134.	308.
Betaine	233.	255.	

SPROUTS, REGENERATION AND NUCLEIC ACIDS

In his article (22) "Make Cells Grow Younger", Brown Landone wrote:

> "More than twenty years ago, experiments were made on old decrepit rats. Their age corresponded to that of a man of ninety years. They were fed with "immature food," that is, food which had not finished growth, sprouting new stems, young leaves. The results were

amazing. The old decrepit rats were transformed, and their bodies began to grow younger . . . Twenty years later, the factor recognized to produce this effect was anxinon (enzymes) . . . The best anxinon foods I know of are produced in mung bean sprouts."

Dr. Weston A. Price isolated in the tips of early grasses a similar substance which promoted healing (23). Rev. Ann Wigmore (48) and Kulvinskas (49) share many healing, rejuvenating experiences produced by immature greens at Hippocrates Health Institute and many other similar research centers.

Dr. Frank, in his clinical study of control and reversal of aging, found that nucleic acids within nuclei of all living cells can have a dramatic effect on aging (139).

Dr. Frank said:

"Basic to the author's approach is the theory that exogenous RNA, especially when combined with metabolically associated B vitamins, minerals, amino acids and sugars, will enter the cell and aid in normal regeneration of the decayed metabolic organization of the cell, and in so doing will bring about normal enzyme synthesis and activation."

Experimental studies "clearly show that exogenous RNA, or related compounds, especially when given along with other metabolites, do indeed visibly reverse aging," Dr. Frank concluded (139).

Nucleic acids are polymers (a substance formed by a combination of two or more molecules of the same substance) of nucleotide (a compound formed of phosphoric acid, sugar and a base).

The best known are ribonucleic Acid (RNA) and deoxyribonucleic acid (DNA). In the DNA we find the master blueprint of living cells controlling heredity and the ability of cells to reproduce. RNA carries the pattern to cells throughout the organism.

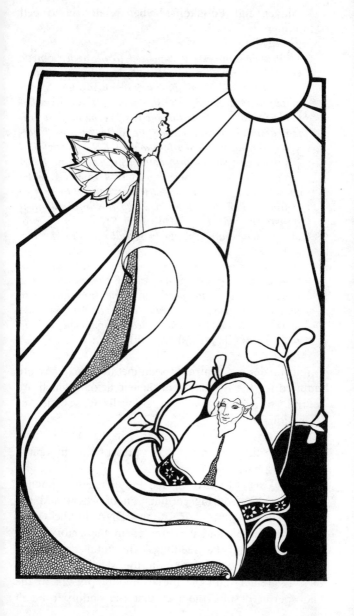

Mayer and Poljakoff-Mayber relates it to cell building:

"*Protein synthesis is supposed to be under genetic control. As proteins are extremely specific in structure it has been suggested that their configuration is ultimately determined by the structure of the deoxyribonucleic acid (DNA) in the nucleus. As the bulk of protein synthesis occurs outside the nucleus in small particles, variously called ribosomes or RNA particles, it is suggested that the information present in the DNA molecule is in some way transferred to RNA molecules, which are more directly associated with protein synthesis. The exact way in which this information is transferred and the way in which RNA controls protein structure and specificity is still open to speculation.*" (3).

"*The nucleic acids constitute an extremely important part of the phosphorus-containing compounds. The nucleic acids occur partly in their free form and partly in the form of nuceoproteins. The ratio of RNA to DNA (ribonucleic acid to deoxyribonucleic acid) in many seeds is approximately 10:1 (3)*".

Phosphates are central to seed metabolism. They are required for the formation of nucleic acids—which are central in protein synthesis as well as genetic information.

Phosphorus in seeds is primarily in the organic form and very little seems to be present as inorganic orthophosphate.

Semenko (141) investigated the changes in nucleic acids occurring during germination of wheat and oat seeds. The amount of RNA and DNA in the endosperm decreased and it increased in the embryo and subsequently in the seedling. The total amount of nucleic acids accumulating in the seedling after 10 days is greater than the initial amount present in the endosperm, despite the fact that the endosperm still contained some nucleic acids. Semenko concludes that nucleic acids are not only transported from the endosperm to the seedling or embryo but are also synthesized de novo in the seedling. Maroti (140) found that in the root both cell number and nucleic acid content rose more quickly than in the shoot.

Dr. Roberts in a study entitled Hydrolyis of some Deoxyribonuclesides by wheat leaf juice (142) identified enzymes that break up RNA into its simpler components making it available for cellular rebuilding.

In conclusion, we state that sprouts have a regenerating effect on the human body because of the high

TABLE 14
Changes In Cell Number And Nucleic Acid Content
Of Beans During Germination
The Numbers Are Per Plant Organ
(Compiled From Maroti, 1957)

Time	Total number of cells		RNA.P.		DNA.P.	
	Root $\times 10^3$	Shoot $\times 10^3$	Root	Shoot	Root	Shoot
6 h	145	66	6.6	1.9	3.0	0.1
1 day	188	80	4.2	1.1	0.9	0.9
2 days	291	104	6.5	4.4	3.3	1.1
3 days	654	193	20.5	4.3	11.0	3.1
4 days	1397	265	26.1	4.3	10.1	4.9
5 days	1316	281	29.8	7.7	30.5	4.9
6 days	1451	431	39.5	12.9	28.3	5.8
7 days	1325	808	—	15.9		7.0
8 days	1298	1383	58.6	18.6	13.1	11.0
9 days	1325	1595	79.1	24.0	3.2	7.5

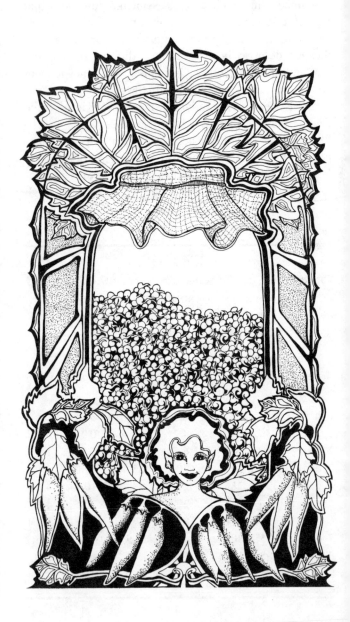

	Time in days	RNA	DNA
wheat	0	2.15	1.02
	2	2.76	1.22
	6	5.76	2.03
	10	7.17	4.85
oat	0	0.97	0.59
	6	1.15	1.38
	10	3.53	1.86

(Semenko, G.I., Fiziol. Rasteny 4,332, 1957)

concentration of RNA, DNA, protein, as well as other essential nutrients which can be found only in a living cell.

SPROUTS AND FERTILITY

Although wheat is one of the highest source of vitamin E, the sprouting process triples total vitamin E content in a period of 3 to 4 days, depending on conditions, so it was reported in Biochemical Journal (36). Sprouted wheat will give you more and better quality vitamin E than found in store bought wheat germ, which is dead food. The minute a seed is split, changes are instigated, which causes the nutrient value to decrease progressively.

The vitamin E (tocopherol) content of dry beans is about the same as in wheat (2.2 mg./100 g.). After few days of sprouting, Benerjee et al (20) noted that beans followed a similar pattern of increase as was observed in "Science" for wheat.

71

TABLE 15

VITAMIN E (TOCOPHEROL) CONTENT SEED (20), MG/100g.

Name	Days of Germination		
	0	2	4
Mung bean	2.4	2.8	3.2
Chickpea	2.0	2.3	2.6
Black bean	1.9	2.4	2.5
Lentil	2.0	2.3	2.1
Green pea	2.2	2.4	1.9

Herting and Emma determined in a set of experiments (28) that the average content of alpha-tocopherol (Vitamin E component) in whole corn, wheat, oat, and rice were 1.53, .87, 1.54 and .35 mg/100g respectively. Up to three-fold variation among samples of the same natural grain was influenced by temperature, soil, and stability after harvest. The processing of grain by flaking, shredding, puffing and other procedures used to produce cereals usually resulted in vitamin E loss up to 90%.

Most foods eaten today contain none, or very little vitamin E, which seems to regulate many important functions of the body, in particular the heart.

Over the years vitamin E has been heralded as the fertility vitamin. Those that want improved virility and return of fertility should include sprouted grains in their diet. Likewise sprouted grains will prevent depletion and earlier disappearance of youth due to sexual practice.

In a Review of Literature Pertaining to the Value of Sprouting Cereal Grains for Livestock Feed: The value of sprouted oats for improving fertility in cattle was studied in several stations. Moore reported results with 4 shy breeders whose rations were supplemented with oat sprouts. Two of the four conceived after having received the supplement. No controls without the supplement were reported. Winters discussed results in which 8 to 10 hard-to-breed cows conceived after being fed 2½ to 5 pounds of sprouted oats for a period of 21 to 90 days. Mosely et al reported five cases in which all conceived at service after initiation of oat sprout supplement. Again no controls were reported. Cunningham reported on conception as the result of supplementing 7 shy breeders with oat sprouts for 70 to 150 days. Miller and Graves reported that 57 of 88 cows conceived within 4 services after oat sprout feeding was started.

Drs. Graves and Miller of the Agriculture Experiment Station at Beltsville, Md. showed the power of sprouts in restoring fertility to sterile cattle. Eleven cows were involved. They had been bred for 6 to 14 months. Three of them were over 8 years old, however they had reproduced successfully in the past. Four were heifers. Each animal was fed 5 pounds of sprouted oat dry weight. The rest of the diet was equal weight of silage. At the end of 60 days, when bred, all cows were made pregnant.

In a bulletin, Dr. J.J. Fayne states:

> *"Tests were made many years ago by the Department of Animal Husbandry of the United States of Agriculture in Beltsville, Maryland, to determine the importance of sprouted oat in restoring fertility. The success was no less than amazing. In every case tested, the cows that had lost or outgrown their ability to reproduce became mothers again, giving birth to fine, normal, healthy calves. The same sprouted grain diet was given to another group of cows that were so completely sterile that they had never reproduced although they had been bred many times. With the addition of nourishment found in these grain sprouts they all became mothers with every evidence of*

healthy reproductive ability. Bulls that had become sterile were also restored to normal fertility again in every case tested. "(The Miracle of Alfalfa)."

Dr. Ehrenfried Pfeiffer, told at Bio-Dynamic Soil Conference in 1951 that "without exception they had never failed to restore to fertility a bull when they have fed him a very limited diet of green alfalfa for a time and then fed generous amounts of sprouted oats." (Three Fold Farm, Spring Valley, N.Y.)

In a 1953 study of unidentified factors relating to reproduction in animals, Kohler (55) found:

1. Feeding of immature grasses to dairy cattle has been shown to increase production of milk.

2. Unidentified water soluble factor in cereal grass juice was found to be effective in producing ovulation of rabbits sensitized with estrogen.

3. An unidentified factor in grass has been reported to produce early vaginal opening and stimulate early ovarian activity in immature rats.

4. Hogan and his co-workers found that green forage contains unidentified nutrients essential to normal reproduction in swine.

5. Wendt found that milk from grass-fed cows, when used by nursing mothers, resulted in the children developing more rapidly than when milk from cows on dry rations was fed.

SPROUT THE FRUIT VEGETABLE

If one is to eat food which is best suited to the physiology then one would have to pick fruit and succulent greens for one's diet. Sprouts are suitable foods for humans. For example, mung beans after 5 days of sprouting become somewhat like a fruit in many ways but appearance. According to Composition of Foods (9) by U.S.D.A. we can make the following observations.

The germination process converts starch to simple

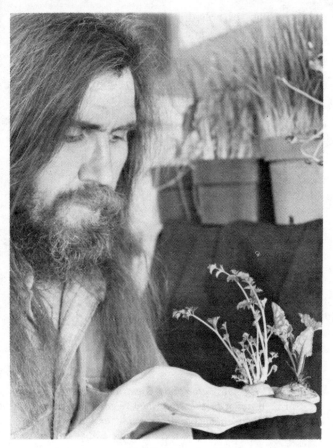

Viktoras 1978

Photo by Ken Olesak

HOW TO SPROUT A CARROT (beet, turnip, parsnip). Cut off ½ inch crown, juice the rest of the carrot. Have a pan with ¼ inch of water. Place the crowns in pan. Add water to pan as needed. In 4 days shoots will develop. In 7 to ten days they can be cut and used in salads. A delicacy. Return the cut crown back to the pan for continued growth. To prevent molding, drain the pan every 2 to 5 days and refill with fresh, cold water.

sugars. The carbohydrate content of the spouted mung bean is the same as you would find in casaba melon. The moisture content increases from 10.7 percent in seed to a value 88.8 percent, comparable to any fruit. The protein concentration is reduced to that of a dry fig. The calorie value is slight, less than that in papaya and a little more than a honeydew melon. Sprouted mung has the vitamin A value of a lemon, thiamin of an avocado, riboflavin of dry apple, niacin of a banana, and ascorbin acid of a pineapple.

I have shown in another book (49) that foods of high mineral composition are not best suited for humans. Sprouting reduces the mineral composition by a factor of two to six of its previous value. Mung sprout has the calcium content of damson plum, potassium level of papaya, sodium concentration of chayote, iron percentage of logenberry (9).

CAN SPROUTS PREVENT CANCER?

Ernest T. Krebs, Jr., biochemist believes that sprouts have anti-cancer factors. He states (44):

> *"Nitrilosides are anti-neoplastic. When they are broken down in the body they release two chemicals. These two chemicals are cyanide and benzaldehyde. Body cells—the normal cells of the body—can protect themselves from such released chemicals, but cancer cells are incapable of doing this . . . both these chemicals kill unprotected cancer cells."*

Krebs continues:

> *"Consider quickly, just the nitriloside content of the diet of primitive man. He relied heavily upon the fresh succulent sprouts of the grasses, the wild legumes, millet, vetch, the lupines, wild beans and the like. Vitamin contents of these plants at the sprouting stage often exceed by 20 times or more that of the*

mature plant. The nitriloside content in the sprouts of some grasses and legumes is often 50 times or more greater than the nitrilosides content of the mature plant. Indeed, the nitrilosides and other accessory food factors that occur in prodigious quantities in the sprouting stage of the plant may be completely absent in the mature plant."

NOISE AND SMOG FREE BEAN

Flatulence plagues mankind, and if it could be channeled to humanitarian ecological usage, it would provide an inexpensive source of fuel in times of crises. From Tom Brown's days at Rugby to the present time, many a school boy has tried his hand at igniting the offending gas to put some light on this clouded scientific mystery. This "Gas crisis" is not a present problem. It has plagued the caveman just as well as the Victorian ladies with their rustling bustles to fan the potential flame. When Mark Twain explored the embarrassing subject on stage in "A Fart in Queen Elizabeth Court", the audience gave a cloudy explosive ovation.

Today the folklore associated with gassing from the musical bean has been under study by U.S. Department of Agriculture near Berkeley, California. They have discovered that a group of complex sugars known as oligo saccharides trigger the creation of the chief gas components. The scientists have found a way to avoid the development of this gas chemistry. They developed a chemical which causes the bean to behave "not as though it is being digested, but as though it is being germinated. For when the bean germinates, it secretes an enzyme called glastosidase, which breaks down the sugars, and thus prevents them from generating the noxious gases of flatulence (45.)"

GRASS, THE EIGHT DAY SPROUT

"All Flesh is grass and its beauty is like the flowers in the field." (Isaiah 40:6).

"One of the most popular of the current health fads is the wheat grass." (Donald C. Healton, Director, U.S. Dept. of Health, Education and Welfare (51).

While living in the suburbs, I discovered that middle-class America is very "grass conscious." There is one measure by which the moral fiber of her citizens is judged—grass, high or low.

A man can cheat on his income tax, take his neighbor's wife to church after a swapping party, default on his credit cards, drink his blue chips away, and the community will forgive him in its heart. But let him fail to keep front lawn mowed and to be seen living in such a field and those forgiving neighborly hearts will turn to stone.

The American front lawn has been sanctioned as a holy place, constantly worshipped but never used. The high priest, the American husband, performs the sacred act of masculinity—the Saturday lawn-mowing rites. On Sunday Mom and Dad enjoy this aesthetic sacrament from the living room. Is there some sort of primitive consciousness that has led to the evolvement of this form of middle-class behavior? Will humans start imitating the morning ritual of their pets?

GRASS POWER

A human's strength is a drop in the bucket compared with that of an elephant, hippopotamus, deer, steer, or horse. Man dies from over 250 diseases, whereas such animals are prone to five or ten diseases. Scientists have no other explanation than that these animals live on a

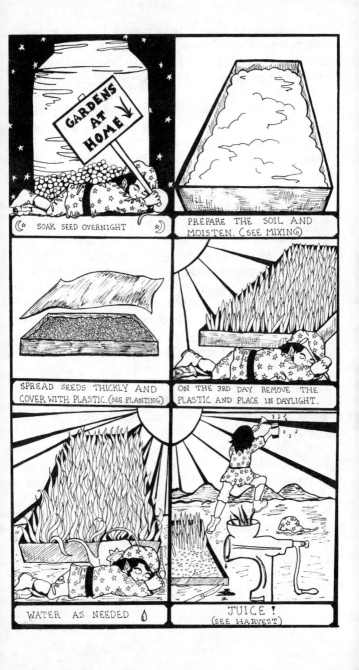

diet produced by nature, not factories (113). We see that humanity could benefit in health by adopting a chlorophyl-rich diet, which includes plenty of wheatgrass and foods rich in all the known nutrients, such as sprouts and fruit.

In the Book of Daniel (94), we recall King Habuchadnezzar, who was a wreck physically and mentally, was advised by heaven to "eat grass as did the oxen." Following the advice, he made a complete recovery.

In the Apocalypse we are told of terrible things to come because we have failed to obey, "and it was commanded that they should not hurt the grasses of the earth, neither any green thing." We have disobeyed by replacing the grasses with highways to make a road for the four galloping horsemen. In Proverbs (19, 12) we are told of the soothing nature of the grass. "The King's wrath is as the roaring of a lion; but his favor is as dew upon the grass." In Jeremiah (14, 6) "Their eyes did fail, because there was no grass."

One of the great researchers in the field of Grasses, Viosin (114) eulogizes the poetry of the pastures: "Few things are able to move us as much as a luxurious meadow standing against a background of dark trees under blue sky. From time immemorial this sight has inspired musicians to translate its beauty into pastoral symphonies. Bathing their eyes in its wonder, painters have presented us with their most beautiful landscape pictures. Green pastures have become the symbol of serenity, of stability, of peace and of plenty. Man's feeling of respect for grass pastures is so profound that he has associated them in his mind with eternal rest, dreaming nostalgically of the green pastures and still waters that await him in the world to come."

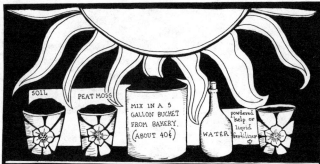

SOIL — PEAT MOSS — MIX IN A 5 GALLON BUCKET FROM BAKERY. (ABOUT 40¢) — WATER — powdered kelp or liquid fertilizer

FOR 1 BAKERS TRAY: 3 HANDFULS OF TOP SOIL, 3 HANDFULS OF PEAT MOSS, AND 1½ QUARTS OF WATER. MIX.

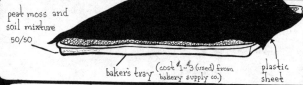

peat moss and soil mixture 50/50

baker's tray (cost $1–$3 (used) from bakery supply co.)

plastic sheet

⬇ PLANTING ALTERNATIVES... ⬇

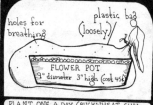

holes for breathing

plastic bag (loosely)

FLOWER POT 9" diameter 3" high (cost 45¢)

PLANT ONE A DAY. (BUCKWHEAT, SUNFLOWER, WHEATGRASS, OR MIXTURE.) SUITABLE FOR ONE OR TWO PEOPLE.

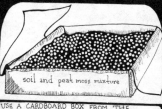

soil and peat moss mixture

USE A CARDBOARD BOX FROM THE GROCERY STORE. USE A 2½" X 3½" GARBAGE BAG AS A LINING AND COVER. (COST 5¢)

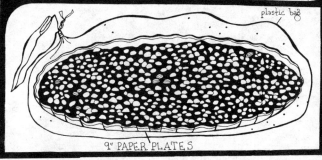

plastic bag

9" PAPER PLATES

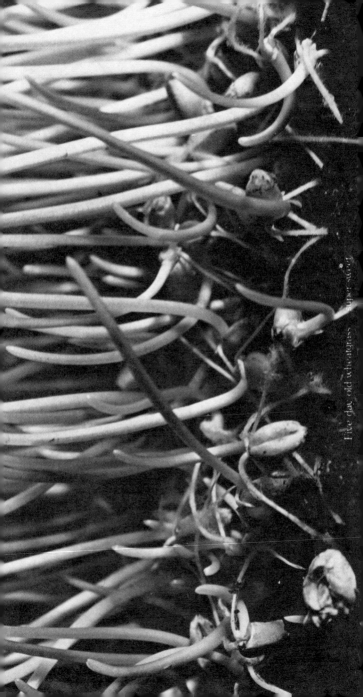

GRASS THE BASIC FOOD

The 1973 issue of the monthly publication "Acres, U.S.A." (115) contains a very informative article on sprouted grain, grass shoots, and grasses, from which we quote:

"WHAT IS A PROTECTIVE FOOD? It is well known that grazing animals can live on grass alone, and pretty poor grass at that. It has been assumed that herbivorous animals could live on any of the common leafy green crops, but this is not the case. A guinea pig is herbivorous, and yet it will die in 8 to 12 weeks on a diet of head lettuce, cabbage or carrots, and will grow at only half its normal rate on a sole diet of spinach. But a guinea pig thrives on a solid diet of grass.

"A super race of guinea pigs was developed in five generations on a sole diet of 20% protein dehydrated grass. The most surprising thing is that a cow could thrive indefinitely on a sole diet of 40% protein grass, yet any farmer knows what would happen to a cow on a sole diet of any concentrate containing 40% protein.

"Grass protein seems to be unique in that it can serve as a source of energy without injuring the liver or kidneys, although this is a wasteful use to make of it. Some new definitions of protein quality are long overdue.

"GRASS AND LIVER FUNCTION. The most notable effect of good grass is the beneficial change it causes in the liver. Not one of 20 leafy green vegetables would cause dark mahogany colored livers which are so conspicuous in grass fed hens. Furthermore, grass fed hens will not approach 100% production until these liver changes take place, but when liver injury has gone far, even good grass won't change or correct the damage.

"Unfortunately, none of the tests for liver function show any sign of liver failure until 90% of the liver has been destroyed, and by that time the victim, either

animal or man, has died of some other degenerative disease, or the liver damage is beyond repair.

"The world has everything but good grass. The ancient shepherd apparently knew that "all flesh is grass", but modern man has had to relearn this homely truth the hard way. These liver changes caused by good grass are too obvious not to have some connection with the prevention of degenerative diseases.

"Dr. F.M. Chidester makes the best summary of the situation from a medical point of view: 'In the early stages of vitamin deficiency, the thyroid gland and other endocrine glands are overactive. This overactivity causes the body to lose enormous amounts of calcium, iodine and iron, which leads to goiter, anemia, nerve degeneration, diabetes, paralysis of the limbs and gastric ulcers. Finally in the later stages of vitamin deficiency, when the glands have become exhausted, sterols accumulate in thebody and form gall stones, cataracts, hardening of the arteries and the most malignant form of cancers. The vitamins of natural foods are best because they have no chemical unbalances.

"Dr. Chidester's theory explains the universal prevalence of tooth decay, even among people getting twice the supposed minimum requirement of calcium. A small amount of good grass in the human diet prevents tooth decay, which is the result of other degenerative changes in the body. Don't ever forget that degenerative diseases start their spiral of destruction before a child is born. Stillbirths are certainly not a NORMAL FUNCTION of motherhood.

"It is folly to dose ourselves with one or two vitamins when we know nothing about their relationship to 50 other food factors. For example, it takes 20% of 20% protein grass to serve as the sole source of vitamins for a guinea pig, but 5% of the grass will fully replace any one vitamin which is purposely left out of a guinea pig's diet. This can only mean that some of the vitamins must be interchangeable with each other. Grass does many things in animal nutrition which

84

cannot be accounted for by its known vitamin content. For example, 40% protein grass is only four to five times as high in known vitamins as 20% of 40% protein grass; it will perform miracles in a poultry ration as compared to 10% of 20% alfalfa grass.

"Either God or man is still mixed up on the subject of vitamins. For example, only man, monkey and the guinea pig are supposed to need Vitamin C. Good grass is the richest natural source of both Vitamin A and Vitamin C, yet grass has been considered fit only for cow feed, and grazing animals are less than 1% efficient in transferring these vitamins to meat, milk and eggs."

GRASS FOR HEALING

One of the first acts cats and dogs perform, after being let out of the home in the morning, is to nibble on some grass. There seems to be some sort of healing, protective property in grass which instinctively makes all classes of animals—carnivorous as well as fruitarian—desire to nibble on the green blade.

A civilized human has only to look in field and forest to learn from the wild animals. They have no hospitals, no doctors, no medicine, yet they are ruled by the same law of creation that governs a human. If a wild animal feels sick, it will nibble on some grass or fast, depending on the instinctual commands of its body.

In America, over 60 percent of the citizens are registered chronically ill, many more are self-medicated. Could that sacred lawn ritual be turned into a true act of worship, for rebuilding the human temple, by making a sacrament of the grass clippings? Would it rejuvenate a sick blubber-drowning American into a nation of healthy youth?

We have been eating fruit of the grass family ever since we left our natural environment. Wheat, rice, corn, bamboo, sugar cane are all members of the grass family. Liver, butter, wheat germ, grass power and yeast are five sources of all the vitamins science has been able to discover and isolate. The source of all five is grass.

A human should not be so prejudiced as to think that just because one has been using grass seed for food for thousands of years that there is something wrong with the grass itself. It is a complete food. It should be included in the diet for both protective and healing value.

GRASS JOINT

In 1931, a young scientist from Kansas, Charles Schnabel, made a significant discovery for the survival of the human race. At the time of forming the first joint, which might be anywhere from 6 to 20 days of growth, vitamin content reaches the highest peak. For this discovery, he obtained a U.S. Patent No. 1,942 on January 9, 1934. Kahler, et al, Department of Agricultural Chemists, University of Wisconsin, reinforced Schnabel's findings. They noted (52) grass is most potent during the period of the most rapid growing stage.

As any child will testify, the grass blade before the first joint is formed is succulent green, sweet and very tasty. Dr. Schnabel, in his pamphlet "Food Buyers Guide" states: "Since grazing animals are parasites on plants, the different families have adopted characteristic methods of protecting themselves from destruction. The trees hold their leaves out of reach. The cactus developed spines. Many plants develop poisons in their leaves.

"But the grasses solved this problem of self-preservation in a way far different from any other family. They joint. All grasses at maturity, like the bamboo fishing pole, have numerous joints or nodes—but it is the formation of the first joint that holds the age-old secret of grass.

"If a grass culm (shoot) is cut or grazed before the first joint forms, it will grow up again, but if cut after that time it will die. This fact has been known for centuries but no significance was ever attached to it till 1913, when it was discovered that: All grass leaves reach a peak of food value, per pound of dry matter, on the day the first joint begins to form."

NUTRIENTS IN GRASS

Dr. A.I. Virtanen (56) and Virtanen and Lane (57) have published a series of papers showing that various green plant constituents reach maximum concentration when plant growth is most rapid. Thus protein, aspartic acid, carotene, and Vitamin C are present in the largest quantities just before the plant reaches the flowering stage.

In Finland, 1938, Dr. A.I. Virtanen published another paper where he showed that cereal grasses reached a high peak of carotene (pro-Vitamin A) on about the 18th day depending on weather conditions. Other vitamins follow a similar pattern. Hunt et al, Record and Beath have shown similar growth patterns of Vitamin B1 and flavin content of pasture grasses and hays, which were correlated with the rate of growth of plants. In reference book, Metabolism (58) we see that wheat grass contains 75,000 I.U. carotene per pound, more than twice the amount found in carrots (59).

Sprague, Crampton and Harris through separate

studies summarized in Metabolism (58) bring out that wheat grass is an excellent source of Calcium, Chlorine, Iron, Magnesium, Phosphorus, Potassium, Sodium, Sulphur, Cobalt and Zinc.

Dr. Burkholder of Yale states that grasses are exceptionally rich source of the B vitamins (37):

> *"Green leaves of young wheat, barley, corn and oats grown outdoors in soil indicated the presence of rich stores of B vitamins in these materials. The thiamine and riboflavin contents of young barley and wheat leaves were particularly striking in comparison with the amounts present in the dry grains. On a dry weight basis there was more than double the amount of thiamine and about 20 times more riboflavin present in the young green leaves than in the dry seed."*

In a private correspondence with Dr. Ann Wigmore, Dr. Earp Thomas of Bloomfield Labs brought out that wheat grass has all the known minerals. However, this is limited by the quality of soil and seed. If seeds grew up for many generations in a depleted soil, a time is reached where the seed will produce a deficient grass. Studies of this subject has been presented by Dr. Voissin (46).

You can anticipate from a kilogram of fresh leaves about 1.5 grams of chlorophyll, while about 7.5 grams can be obtained from a kilo of dried leaves (71). Dr. Earp Thomas of Bloomfield Labs, New Jersey, in a private communication to Dr. Ann Wigmore, asserted that wheat grass is one of the highest sources of chlorophyll. In a study (72) of wheatgrass grown under a light intensity of 1,000 foot candles, under varied photoperiods of 0 to 24 hours, Dr. Wolf of the Department of Biology, Vanderbilt University, Nashville, Tenn., discovered that chlorophyll content reached a maximum value of .9 mg/gram in a 20 hour photoperiod.

The following is an analysis by the Wisconsin Alumni Research Foundation of the composition of oat grain and oat grass, dried after 5 days of growth. We can note that all the nutrients increase over the values found in the dry seed. The same pattern follows for all other grasses:

TABLE 16

CONSTITUENTS (%)	GRAIN	GRASS
Dry Matter	100	100
Protein	15	21
Ether Extract (fat)	4.21	5.2
Nitrogen Free Extract	65.86	42.79
Fiber	11.71	26.11
Ash	3.22	3.9
Calcium	.063	.238
Phosphorus	.360	.509
Carotene (mg)	0.	39.067
Vitamin E (mg)	17.95	48.87
Riboflavin (mg)	1.96	22.29
Thiamin (mg)	3.14	12.86
Niacin (mg)	7.18	103.96
Vitamin C (I.U.)	0.	4366.5

E.E. Pfeiffer, in a study (61), "Protein Changes During Germination and Earliest Leaf Growth," grew grain hydroponically—using air, water and compost. He showed that on the 7th day the highest protein value of the wheatgrass reaches 4.8 percent of the total leaf. At that time, it is 89% moisture. By the time it reaches the 8th day of growth, it has also developed lysine, one of the essential amino acids, which is absent at earlier stages of growth.

In other studies (49), I brought out the benefit of low protein diet. It is interesting that according to Pfeiffer (61), if one dehydrates the grass, the protein composition can be as high as 47.4 percent. Some farmers have noted that hay, dried grass, fed in too liberal a quantity, will make the animals sick. It is too much protein. Dried wheatgrass has three times as high a protein concentration as steak, but wheatgrass juice only one-third the protein concentration of beef. Hence, wheatgrass juice is suitable for man, but not dehydrated grass preparation unless in very diluted form.

All animals obtain their basic nutrition, directly or indirectly, from a grass. Through recorded history, the use of fresh green grass as a basic feed for livestock has revealed the vital need for year-round feeding of its life-giving juices. Dr. George D. Scarseth, Director of Research of the American Farm Research Association, West Layfayette, Indiana, says: "Somewhere in the food chain of all people something green was the starting point."

Dr. George C. Kohler of Cerophyl Laboratories, Inc. in Kansas City, has reported that although it will be many years before the chemical nature and physiological importance of the unidentified factors in grass are fully known, it is essential that adequate amounts be included in livestock and poultry rations.

He pointed out in terms of animal or human requirements as compared to other natural sources—green leaf products are very rich in Vitamin A activity, ascorbic acid, Vitamin E, Vitamin K and thiocitic acid. In addition to the "identified vitamins, green vegetation is an excellent source of a variety of unidentified vitamins," Dr. Kohler stated. The GRASSES are NON-TOXIC in any usable amount. Experiments at Kansas City University as partially written up in FEDERATION PROCEEDINGS, Vol. 15, No. 1, March 1956 (article No. 33, page 11) being the official annual magazine of six scientific organizations, showed that doses were used on laboratory rats equivalent in humans to 500 tablets daily of 7 grains each, being a 45-day supply taken daily.

In a recent publication in the Journal of Nutrition (52, 53, 54) results were presented to show that various supplements rich in the known vitamins produced little or no growth response in rats on basal winter milk diet. This led to the conclusion that the growth-stimulating factor was distinct from all known vitamins.

In another experiment rats were fed on mineralized winter milk adlibitum plus a variety of supplements while their weight and general health was observed. Kohler found growth and health stimulated by 3 gm fresh grass, 3 cc grass juice, and .6 gm dried oats grass. Inferior growth response was produced by daily doses of 2 drops of cod liver oil, 1 cc orange juice, .5 gm brewer's yeast, .25 gm dried brain and 1.0 gm defatted wheat germ.

In a later experiment (54), Kohler et al used the herbivorous guinea pigs. He fed them mineralized winter milk plus supplements containing liberal quantities of known vitamins. Brewer's yeast, orange juice and liver extracts effected an inferior response. The remarkable growth produced by supplementing grasses adds credence to the hypothesis that the "grass juice factor" described for rats is the same factor concerned in this later experiment.

Kohler showed that wheat and barley grass was most effective in producing a growth rate. It offset the normal weight loss (and eventual death) which was shown to set in on a pasteurized milk diet. It was noted that extracted juice contains the active factor for both rats and guinea pigs, and the activity of the grasses disappeared upon storage at room temperature.

What was really surprising, as Kohler states: "The animals receiving mineralized milk, orange juice and

91

grass juice grew at good rates and no abnormalities were observed. When the grass juice was omitted, the animals died."

Dr. W. R. Graham of Ontario, Canada, worked on "gray hair factor" in grass research. He found black mice got gray hair if they were denied grass vitamins.

In "Feeds and Feeding", Frank B. Morrison writes that green forage crops not only supply most of the vitamins which have been discovered thus far, but also furnish other unknown vitamins. Farm animals suffer from nutritive deficiencies when never allowed on pasture or fed fresh, green forage. Even the best of hay is not a substitute for green feed. In reviews of Grass Juice Investigation by G.O. Kohler, it is pointed out that a water soluble growth factor in grass has been found to be required for optimum growth of chicks, turkeys and geese.

How do we know that a forage juice contains an unidentified growth factor? Where chicks were fed a ration complete in protein, minerals and all vitamins, they grew at a reasonably good rate. Adding 3 percent of forage juice concentrate caused an increase in growth rate of 5 to 15%. Adding higher levels of all known vitamins including inositol, choline, ascorbic acid and all the B vitamins did not have any effect on the growth rate.

M.L. Scott's work, "The Grass Juice Factor in Turkey Nutrition," states the need by poults for unidentified factors in grass. The experiments showed that the factors were not stable during storage. Supplementation of the feed with 5% of fish meal in addition to the 5% already present in the basal diet produced no increase in poult growth. Whereas, 5% fresh grass juice promoted a marked gain over that of the poults receiving basal diet.

While mature grass is an excellent source of the growth factor, dehydrated grass contains little or none,

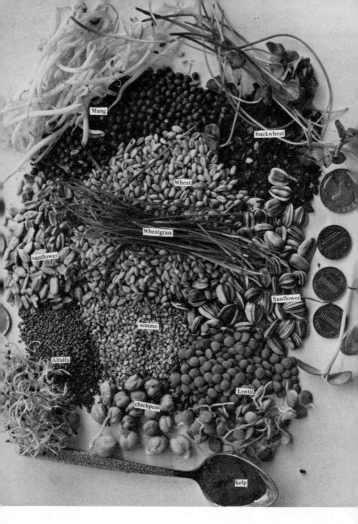

Meal For Famine or Feast

indicating that the unknown factor is either destroyed or rendered unavailable to the poult during processing. However, immature grass (less than ten days old), dehydrated under low temperature, does have the growth factor (116).

The amount of the factor varied with the age of the plant, excellent concentration being present in the growing plant, while the mature and old plant contained considerably less. Hydrogen peroxide treatment destroyed practically all the activity, including the destruction of the grass juice factor to be an oxidative process.

Work at Cornell has shown that the forage factor deficiency is usually the first limiting factor for growth of poults. The turkey poult studies showed that dehydration destroyed most of the growth factor. Also, it was shown that juice from grasses was equivalent in activity to alfalfa juice.

For additional details on the grass juice factor see also U.S. Government "Yearbook of Agriculture 1959" page 165.

When grass juice is utilized for human nutrition, we see that it is advisable to use the grass immediately after harvesting, unless it is stored under refrigeration. Even there you can anticipate losses. Furthermore, the juice should be extracted either by chewing or utilizing a slow action machine. Centrifugal juicers and blenders are not suited, because the fast rotation oxidizes the grass juice.

GRASS FOR SURVIVAL

In time of emergency, a nation can recognize an unusual, easily accessible food source. "England is prepared to use grass for food if supplies run low," said Professor John B. Johnstone Wallace of Cornell University during World War II. He reported to the Canadian Institute of Public Affairs in 1942 that the production of grass is in operation and is being tested on animals. He added, "It will soon be fed to human beings if they are wise." Johnstone-Wallace has used grass himself, mixed half and half with flour and baked in soda biscuit. He said "Green grass is nutritious and tastes real fine."

Dr. Charles Schnabel, formerly of Rockhurse College, Kansas City, declared that: "the time is not far off when we will be consuming a daily portion of grass in butter, bread, milkshakes, candy bars, breakfast foods, pancakes and even ice cream and cookies."

At one point in her development Dr. Moore-Pataleena of London, England said: "I have been eating grass for six years and I'm getting younger every day. When the grass is tender, I eat it whole; if it is tough I extract the juice." Dr. Moore, at one-time a chronically sick woman, after completing her 1,028 mile hike across England, started a 3,200 mile walk across America. Asked what she would use for fuel, she replied "Grass."

Dr. Ann Wigmore, founder of the Hippocrates Health Institute, in the publication Rising Sun (48) which reaches over 40 countries, has for years advocated the use of grass and live foods for therapeutic purposes. As a young woman, she had gangrene in both of her legs. She cured herself through the use of grass. Later she found grass to be an effective in treating all chronic disorders.

Ann Wigmore, in one of her publications reflects on the history of wheat, writes: "Some 120 centuries ago, on the continent of Atlantis, which later sank beneath the sea, it was predicted that the real health properties of wheat would not be learned until some far distant future generation were given the key which would save a tottering civilization from extinction." We are such a generation. Wheatgrass could be the tool for regaining health.

Charles Schnabel likens the necessity of the X factor in grass to the childhood poem, "The House That Jack Built" in the rhyme, "The Eskimo ate the seal that ate the fish that ate the kelp (sea grass) that lived in the sea that 'ate' the sun from the sky and the minerals in the sea that came from the streams that drained the soil where the rocks weathered." We eat the steak or drink the milk that comes from the cow that eats the grass.

The few so-called experts may discount the importance of the grass juice factor in human nutrition, but those drinking grass juice through these critical times will be better prepared to survive the ecological crises. Scientific work will continue, and more specific facts about grass will appear. However, we can take advantage now of the "x factor" in grass juice and feel the difference in our sense of strength, health, spirituality, endurance and well being.

CHLOROPHYLL → *builds* hemoglobin

For ages men have puzzled over the question— "What makes grass green?" About a century ago chemists suggested the green pigment in growing plants and named it chlorophyll.

A certain belief evolved about this green fluid. The fact that herbivora build hemoglobin (blood cell pigment) on a diet composed of leafy greens invites the hypothesis that derivatives of chlorophyll may be used in making hemoglobin. A. Dr. Abderhalden in his text book (63) suggest that blood pigment might be made from plants.

Added to this biological relationship is the chemical similarity between chlorophyll and hemoglobin. This was suggested by Verdeil (64) in 1851, though on the basis of invalid evidence. It was substantiated in 1789 by Hoppe-Seyler (65) who showed a similarity between hematin and chlorophyll derivatives.

Willstater's work (66) between 1906 and 1913 identified chlorophyll as an unstable water soluble magnesium compound characterized by ester groups of methyl and phytyl alcohol. He further showed (67) both chlorophyll and hemoglobin to be closely related, both had some phyrrole fragments.

The years of research that were stimulated by Verdel's hypothesis culminated in the series of brilliant investigations by Hans Fisher, for which he was awarded the Nobel Prize in 1930 (68). He and his co-workers finally established the correct structure of hemin, part of the hemoglobin, by synthesis, and showered the true relationship to chlorophyll.

They observed that the chlorophyll molecule closely resembles hemin, the pigment which when combined with protein, forms hemoglobin. The latter is present in the red corpuscles of the blood and by carrying oxygen to the tissues makes the production of energy and life feasible.

One of the major differences between chlorophyll and hemin is that chlorophyll contains magnesium while hemin molecule contains iron for the central atom (69). Note, hemoglobin is one of the most important constituents of cells, it makes up three quarters of the solid content (70).

GREENS HEAL ANEMIA

Owing to the close molecular resemblance between chlorophyll and hemoglobin, it was believed by Frans Miller, another scientist, that chlorophyll is nature's blood-building element for all plant eaters and humans. He writes: "Chlorophyll has the same fast blood-building effect as iron in animals made anemic." This has led also to a great deal of controversy.

What exactly is anemia? According to Webster's dictionary, anemia is a condition in which there is a reduction of the number of red blood corpuscles or the total amount of hemoglobin in the blood stream or both. Thus anemia is an excellent vehicle for the study of the relationship between food and hemoglobin count.

The first scientist to demonstrate the regenerative effect of chlorophyll on animals was Dr. Emil Burgi (73) who in 1916 observed that rabbits rendered anemic by bleeding recovered more rapidly when chlorophyll was added to their diet.

Scott (75) showed that a diet of milk, white bread and chlorophyll rebuilt blood faster than bread and milk. Scott and Delor noted (74) that iron-and-copper-free alfalfa extract relieved milk induced anemia.

Patek and Minor (78) in clinic study with rare type anemia caused by pigment scarcity, observed a small positive increase in hemoglobin concentration on intravenous injection of chlorine derivative. Dr. Fisher in Germany announced that for some time he had been using chlorophyll in the treatment of anemia with promising (although by no means conclusive) results (79).

In another clinic study Dr. Patek (76) used fifteen adult patients with chronic hypo-chronic anemia. They were given chlorophyll and allied substances, and were placed on house diets free of meat and eggs, whereas the diet was adequate in all other respects. The Crude chlorophyll was a tar-like substance extracted from alfalfa leaves. It was found that chlorophyll alone was not effective. When chlorophyll and its derivatives were administered there was an increase in hemoglobin and the improvement in the sense of well being.

Other workers have reported curative effects of chlorophyll and its derivatives in a wide variety of anemias: protein deficiency (77), hemorrhagic (80, 86), phenyl hydrazine poisoning (82,83), pernicious (77,84) hypochronic of unknown etiology (76) and "experimental nutritional anemia" of unidentified character (85). Some of the reports are based on clinical studies, while others are the results of animal experimentation.

J. Howell Hughes and A.L. Latner from the Department of Physiology, University of Liverpool, in his highly discriminative experiment, (86) finally resolved the question of blood regeneration capacity of chlorophyll. Rabbits were made anemic by daily bleeding, reducing the hemoglobin level to two fifths of the normal value. The rabbits were split into two groups. The experimental received in diet chlorophyll in oil, the control only oil.

They performed five experiments. Three with varying degrees of pure chlorophyll, one with large doses of crude chlorophyll (unrefined), one with magnesium-free chlorophyll derivatives. The following is a summary:

1. Pure chlorophyll in large doses has no effect on the speed of hemoglobin regeneration after hemorrhage. It seems large doses are toxic to the bone marrow.

2. Very small doses of pure chlorophyll markedly increased the speed of hemoglobin regeneration to approximately its previous level.

3. Crude chlorophyll is effective even in large doses.

Hughes concludes: "It seems therefore that the animal body is capable of converting chlorophyll to hemoglobin." This is in agreement with Zin (87) who, however, showed the effect of chlorophyll injection on the red blood cell count of animals not rendered anemic.

Thus we see how chlorophyll can aid in rebuilding the bloodstream. Without correcting all the causes of anemia, the chlorophyll results are temporary in nature and not consistently workable with every individual. If, however, the individual was to be placed on organic live foods and on one of the richest crude forms of chlorophyll then the results are always the same, and the anemic condition disappears. Rev. Ann Wigmore (47, 48) in clinical studies has proven this many times.

CHLOROPHYLL AND LIGHT

It is interesting to note that chlorophyll absorbs energy from the sun and in some unknown way uses it for the manufacture of sugar, starch and proteins (88). Lois Miller describes (79) poetically the process:

> "A ray of sunshine strikes the green leaf and instantly the miracle is wrought. Within the plant molecules of water and carbon dioxide are torn apart—a feat which the chemist can accomplish with a great deal of difficulty and expense. First there are only lifeless gas and water; then presto! These elements are transformed into living tissue and useful energy. Oxygen is released from the plant to revitalize the air we breathe. Units of energy, in sugar and other carbohydrates, are speedily manufactured and stored up in living plant."

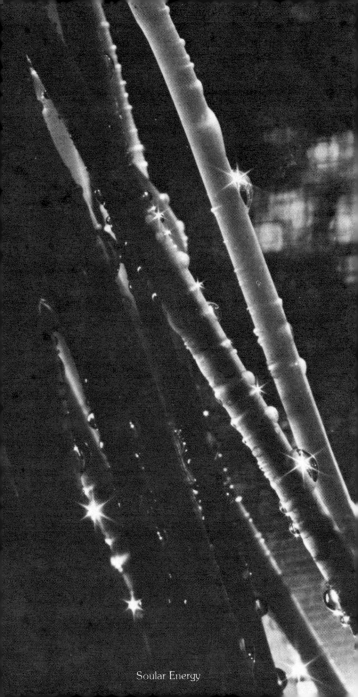
Soular Energy

It is possible, a similar miraculous technology is being exercised in the more pliable mobile brothers by their hemoglobin structure. Emma Dietz (89) of Harvard University ponders the irony. "In the slow development of the chemistry of these two pigments, it has been an increasing source of wonder to chemists to find two substances of such widely different origin and function, and yet so remarkably similar in structure."

Is it possible—such a discrepancy between structure and function? I believe it is not! If hemoglobin exercised only a limited number of functions in transporting oxygen from the lungs to the tissue, we would not find so many secondary favorable side effects in all forms of chronic disorders when treated with chlorophyll sources.

My belief is that the hemoglobin in the body of a perfectly balanced individual can keep body together and health indefinitely, by converting the solar radiation into the essential nutrients. The thousands of individuals in recorded history who lived for years without any food give weight to this argument. One of the recent examples, Teresa Newman, a Catholic Saint, who died about five years ago, lived for 20 years without food or water. Her home had a glass roof, as she realized her dependence on solar radiation and the light of God. (117, 49).

CHLOROPHYLL AND CHRONIC DISEASES

The widescale effect on chronic disorders of chlorophyll, ranging from skin infections to cancer, have been recorded in many medical journals. I will scratch only the surface, in describing some of the research.

In July 1940 (79) the first comprehensive report on

the therapeutic use of chlorophyll was published in the American Journal of Surgery. Under these auspices, and with testimonials of many distinguished doctors, the green pigment was described as an important and effective drug.

Some 1,200 cases, ranging from deep internal infections like brain ulcer and peritonitis to skin disorders and pyorrhea, had been treated and documented, and in case after case the doctors had been able to close their reports with: "Discharged as cured."

People had been brought into the hospital with bursting or infected appendix and spreading peritonitis. Appendectomies had been performed, and the task of checking the gravely dangerous infection was done with chlorophyll. They flooded the deep wounds through drainage tubes with chlorophyll solution, and applied it elsewhere on wet dressing or in ointments and salves.

Ulcerated varicose veins, osteomyelitis (a difficult bone infection), skin disorders and various types of infected wounds have been cured and healed. Applied in numerous cases of mouth infections, such as Vincent's angina and advanced pyorrhea, the results were immediate and positive. "The gums tightened up entirely," Dr. H.D. Junkin commented, and have remained clean since.

The most spectacular results occurred in the treatment of chronic sinus infections and head colds. Of the 1,000 cases of respiratory infections—sinusitis, rhinitis, head colds, etc.,—treated under supervision of Drs. R. Ridpath and T.C. Davis, prominent specialists, "there is not a single case recorded in which either improvement or cure has not taken place." Chlorophyll packs inserted into the sinuses had a drying effect, clearing up congestion, and gave immediate relief . . . Congested head colds were cleared up within 24 hours.

Other teams of specialists reported just as favorable results. Dr. Burgi (90) and his co-workers use chlorophyll in the treatment of anemia, tuberculosis, cardiac disease, arteriosclerosis and mental depression because of its "tonic" effect.

The efficiency of chlorophyll as a tissue stimulant and healing agent in case of tropic ulcer, varicose ulcers, decubitus ulcers, pilonidal cysts, osteomyelitis, and other conditions of topical application has been proven by Bowers (91), Morgan (92) and Boehme (93). Furthermore, Doctors at Temple University in Philadelphia discovered (79) that the green solution seems to thicken and strengthen the body cell walls of living animals.

Smith and Livingston (94) produced experimental surgical wounds in 1372 animals, and found that chlorophyll reduced the healing period by 25% in more than two thirds of the cases compared with controls.

Drs. Bertham and Weinstock (95) said: "Our evidence suggests that the method of treatment (chlorophyll, urea, benzocaine) described will materially reduce the period of disability (infected corns, ingrown nails, calluses and tape reactions) and avoid the possibility of reaction that might otherwise occur from the use of systematic antibiotics."

Gruskin (96) reported the deodorizing and tissue stimulating effect of local applications of chlorophyll.

Offenkrantz reported (97) the following study. A total of 79 patients with X-ray proved duodenal and **gastric ulcers** were treated with powder incorporating water-soluable chlorophyll, "Coating" material and recognized antacid. **The treatment was not accompanied with the usual restriction on diet, smoking, alcoholic beverages or daily activity.**

Of the group, **58 showed on roentgenelogical examination complete healing** in two to seven weeks; 60 experienced complete symptomatic relief in from one to three days.

Of the 27 patients which had a peptic ulcer of long duration previous to the chlorophyll treatment, the majority of those cases had undergone treatment with accepted therapies incorporating strict diets, antacids, aluminum gels and mucin preparations.

In 20 out of the 27 cases the pain and the other subjective symptoms disappeared with regularity in 24 to 72 hours after treatment started. No toxicity was encountered. Of 24 patients examined with X-rays after treatment, 20 showed complete healing in two to seven weeks of treatment. There was no occurrence of symptoms of the cases showing complete healing, which were followed for periods of from 4 to 11 months.

Boehme (93) reported **over 50 cases of chronic leg ulcers** which had a high percent of rapid healing. Many of these cases were unhealed **from one to eight years** but obtained complete healing by chlorophyll therapy in three to ten weeks. Carpenter (98), Carleson and Garsten (100), and Juul-Moller and Mikkolsen (99) reported similar success with chronic ulcer and osteomyelitis.

Drs. Rafsky and Krieger reported (101) a case study of twenty patients with colon disorders of whom 11 had **ulcerative colitis.** "The methods of treatment which were employed were as follows: **Rectal installation** of various dilutions of chlorophyll solution as retention enema once daily . . . patient instructed to retain fluid as long as possible. No evidence or irritation resulted from the treatment and the solution as a rule was retained for several hours. When the patients began to improve, they were able to retain the chlorophyll solution overnight . . . Definite improvement was seen in the majority of cases."

Rev. Ann Wigmore (47) has advocated such an implanting procedure for all chronic disorders. By laying down on an incline, with the colon raised above the chest, the wheatgrass chlorophyll juice resides in the colon where it is absorbed in twenty to forty minutes. Most sick individuals have decomposing matter residing

105

in the colon from many years of wrong diet. This is one of the primary causes of disease. The implants help to remove this matter and bring back vitality to the eliminative organ. The implant is proceeded by at least 2 enemas to clean out the colon.

Drs. F. Paloscia and G. Polloteen (102) use chlorophyll therapy with some success in the treatment of tuberculosis empyema. Cancer (53, 54, 55) patients seem to have benefited to some degree from chlorophyll therapy, although the results are inconclusive.

Dr. Edmond Fowler reported (70) in 1950 favorable side effects in the use of chlorophyll and mixture: "It should be noted that most of these patients in addition to an improvement in hearing and a lessening of tinnitus (ringing sound in the ear) also improved in general health as well as relief from a variety of other symptoms. There were no undesirable side effects. For what it may be worth although most were older people none have suffered a coronary."

CHLOROPHYLL IS SAFE

Can there be such a beneficial tonic that can still be considered safe without side reactions? Toxicity studies (71, 91, 101) have shown that chlorophyll is absolutely non-toxic when administered parentally (intravenously or intramuscular) or by mouth in animals and humans.

Drs. Hughes and Latner (86) from their experiment using oral dosage of pure and crude chlorophyll discovered: Very small dosages of pure chlorophyll exerted a favorable effect on blood regeneration; however in large dosages it is toxic to the bone marrow. In the case of crude chlorophyll, large doses exerted a favorable effect on hemoglobin regeneration.

Wheatgrass juice is a crude chlorophyll and can be

taken orally or as an implant without worry of toxic side effects. Nature always provides what is safe for humans.

Dr. Lawrence Smith (71), professor of Pathology, reports in his study on the effect of water-soluble chlorophyll preparations on cultures of a variety of the more common pathogenic bacteria. The results tend to support the premise that chlorophyll acts to produce an unfavorable environment for bacterial growth rather than by any direct action upon the bacteria themselves.

CHLOROPHYLL AND BREATH

Rapp and Gurney, as quoted by Offenkrantz (97), at Loyola University established that **water soluble chlorophyll inhibits the action of proteolitic bacteria** (which break down of protein into simpler substances) and enzymes. Hence when taken internally, via mouth or rectum, it inhibits the **putrefaction of protein by some of the bacteria that are commonly found in the digestive track of meat eaters.**

In all these reports, there seems to be general agreement that chlorophyll is bacteriostatic and that the wound-healing property is due to the stimulation of tissue granulation. They all indicate that water-soluble chlorophyll is bland and non-toxic.

Wescott concerned himself with the effect of ingested chlorophyll on the body and breath odors. He says it is effective in neutralizing obnoxious odors in the mouth from foods, beverages, tobacco and metabolic changes (halitosis). It effectively neutralized obnoxious odors from perspiration due to physical exercise, nervousness, etc., obnoxious foot odors, menstrual odors and many urine odors, all the result directly, or indirectly, of the food eaten, especially of meat origin.

The chlorophyll used for neutralizing odors is water

soluble. The natural oils have been removed. When chlorophyll is taken in form of vegetarian diet, it is freed only to a limited extent from the encased walls of the vegetable cells and consequently little is absorbed. This answers the question why goats have such obnoxious odor when they eat grass all the time.

When juice is extracted from the grass, the chlorophyll is released, and for those that need it for body odors it can act as an effective agent. But body odors are the signs that all is not well in an individual. A change in diet, grass juice and a short fast would clear it up.

From this presentation, it is quite evident that chlorophyll, with and without any additional dietary changes can have a great effect on a wide range of disorders. Total, consistent healing would be observed by the medical doctors, if, in addition to their approach, they eliminated the causes, instead of attempting to make the symptoms disappear. In the majority of cases the problems are dietary in nature and unless some drastic changes are made in diet, the symptoms will reappear at some later date.

GREEN, THE ANTI-RADIATION FACTOR

Considerable evidence is being accumulated which indicates that a chlorophyll-rich diet can affect the survival of experimental animals undergoing lethal doses of radiation. In 1950, Lourou and Lartigue (81) reported that cabbage supplement increased the resistance of guinea pigs to radiation. Further studies by Duplan (106) with cabbage, Spector and Colloway (107) with broccoli, and Colloway et al (108) with broccoli and alfalfa indicated that certain plants may reduce the effect of radiation on guinea pigs.

In the experiment, every animal which has received no greens died within 10 to 15 days, while mortality among the green eaters was only about half as great during the same period. So when they start dropping bombs, take some wheatgrass to your shelter, you might even survive. In our daily contact, we are exposed to all sort of radiation sources, and chlorophyll rich foods should be included as part of the protective living.

WHEATGRASS & FLUORIDE

In a private communication on December 6, 1961 to Dr. Ann Wigmore from Bloomfield Laboratories, High Bridge, New Jersey, Dr. Earp-Thomas confirmed the efficiency of chlorophyll-rich wheat grass in neutralizing the toxicity of sodium fluoride, which is a rat poison and is used in the fluoridation of drinking water. He said: "Fluorine rapidly combines with calcium phosphate and other kinetic elements to lose its toxic properties, and harden teeth and bones. That is why fresh grass would act like a catalyst to speedily change the acid fluorine into a beneficial component with a positive reaction. By using wheatgrass, which is comparatively rich in calcium phosphate, it would remove any free fluoric acid and its negative charge to an alkaline calcium phospate fluoride combination with a positive reaction."

Can so beneficial a tonic be completely safe, without side reactions? From toxicity studies we have seen that crude chlorophyll is absolutely non-toxic when administered to animals or humans. Why not use it?

CAN SCIENCE KNOW WHAT
GOD PUT INTO LIFE?

Analysis can serve no nutritional function outside of providing some degree of reassurance that the food may be rich in certain identified nutrients. Intellectually, such analysis might be quite satisfying; besides, it keeps many nutritionists and biologists off welfare lines. But practically it serves very little purpose. No scientist could structure a synthetic diet, then feed an animal and expect it to stay alive on such a diet.

It reminds one of "Humpty Dumpty" who had a great fall and all the king's men couldn't put Humpty together again. Today, the nutritionists are faced with the same dilemma; technology has shattered mother earth's foods, but nutritionists cannot find all the needed pieces to feed us.

Henry C. Sherman, Prof. of Chemistry, Columbia University states: "The chemist could analyze most foods with as near an approach to 100% as he could analyze most other natural things; but could not maintain normal nutrition by feeding the food constituents which his analysis reveals (151)."

We know that the nutritional content is dependent on the genetic history of seed and on fertilizer, rainfall, seasonal temperature, sun spot cycle, electromagnetic storms, pollution, prayer, human aura, bioactivity of soil, composition of soil, etc. We have identified to date only several hundred nutritionally significant components. However, the research continues to point out that each newly discovered micronutrient can have a long-term effect if it is missing in diet. A classic study was done by Prof. Voisin (46) to illustrate this point.

The conclusion one draws is that by eating raw, natural, organic foods which are supplemented with sea or land grasses, weeds and sprouts we can be assured of

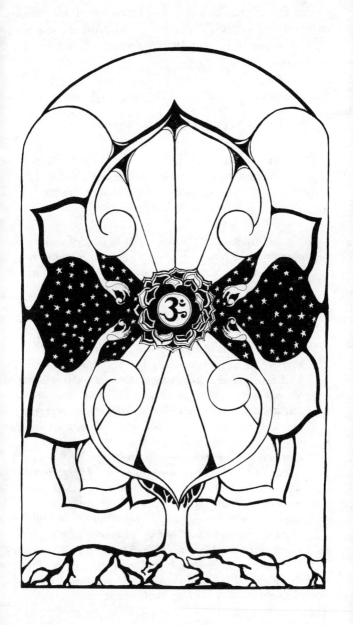

eating an optional diet that will protect us from malnutrition and ecological poisoning and provide us with all known nutrients, plus all those which are yet to be discovered.

TESTING OF LIVE FOOD

Dr. Ann Wigmore received a letter from Harvey Lisle, a chemist, which was in part reproduced in her book SPIRITUAL DIET (144), which reads as following:

> *"Unfortunately the testing of food is destructive of the life in the food. To give several examples: In protein testing the plant tissue is boiled in strong sulfuric acid; in carotene testing the plant tissues are permeated with chloroform and acetone. So it goes with all chemical food testing.*
>
> *The ultimate testing of any food would be the effect upon the human being who ate it. This is almost impossible to do because people vary widely in age, health, metabolic functioning, etc. For this reason biochemists resort to small animal testing. The small test animals have a number of advantages over humans. Their generation span can be measured in weeks or months, whereas for the human being the generation is approximately 70 years.*
>
> *The Haughly Farm, now called the Pye Research Foundation, in England, is the most famous organic farm in the world. After over 25 years of testing their food products in a chemical laboratory, they instituted a small animal testing program which gave much more reliable answers than the chemical testing. We have come full circle and now must go back to small animal testing for the results we want. This is the only way to test living food.*

Natural Cereal Grains vs. Commercial Granola—
When grains are cracked, rolled or shredded their life is destroyed. The protective sheath is destroyed and the contents are subject to oxidation—a life-destroyer. Several serious disadvantages accrue quickly. The oil inherent in the grain begins to oxidize and thereby becomes suspect of becoming a carcinogen. For this reason the broken grains in commercial granolas should be kept sealed and refrigerated as well as possible. Rancidity is nothing more than oxidized oils, and commercial granolas can and do become rancid. Another disadvantage in the broken grains of commercial granolas is the loss of the enzyme activity. We know that one of the advantages of sprouting grains is the activation of their enzyme system. By utilizing sprouted grains in a home-prepared granola, the tremendous boost of the enzyme system is activated.

Isolation of Vitamins—*Nature does not produce a food product with just Vitamin A or Vitamin D or any other individual vitamin in it. Rather, nature produces a balance of vitamins in each of her many food products. Vitamins may be likened to an orchestra which is composed of many musical instruments all working in concert. For example, an apple or carrot or parsley would have many vitamins in them all working together.*

To take an individual vitamin such as Vitamin C violates the law of Nature. Nature produces no food product that contains only Vitamin C. Fortunately, the person taking Vitamin C, for example, is supplementing it with the naturally-occurring vitamins in his or her food.

There has been more research work done on vitamins than any other component of food and yet the basic facts of vitamins are almost lost by both the researchers and laymen.

It is necessary to recognize "living forces" as separate and apart from materialistic concepts. It is impossible to analyze or separate out vitamins. Vitamins are something immaterial, a "living force." Foods rich in vitamins such as wheat grass or carrots take in the living forces so that the living forces are integral with the wheat grass and carrots and cannot be separated out.

What is the main source of this living force? The main source is the sun. We think of the sun's rays as light rays but in reality many different types of rays come into the world from the sun which are not visible to us. The infra-red rays and ultra-violet rays are examples.

Foods rich in Vitamin A are those rich in "warmth" such as oils and seeds. Warmth is derived from the sun—mostly from the infra-red rays of the sun.

Foods rich in Vitamin B are those rich in "order" such as the husks of wheat berries or rice and the peels of fruit. Order derives from the ultra-violet rays of the sun.

Foods rich in Vitamin C are those rich in "light" such as green leaves (like wheat grass). Light derives from the visible rays of the sun.

Vitamin D is in another category. The best way to describe Vitamin D is to relate an experiment with pigeons which had their oil glands under their tails removed. They developed rickets, the disease associated with Vitamin D deficiency. When preening their feathers, the pigeons could no longer oil their feathers so that the sun could irradiate the oil into Vitamin D followed by absorption of the irradiated oil into the bird's skin. Undoubtedly our best Vitamin D source is the Vitamin D we ourselves can properly absorb through our skin from the rays of the sun. My personal practice is to expose a reasonable amount of my skin to the sun whenever conveniently possible.

Paradoxically, the warmth, light and air which impart the "living forces" to growing foods will destroy them after they have been harvested. Take hay, for example, which is livestock's chief source of complete vitamins. A farmer will store his hay, protecting it as much as possible from light, heat and moving air currents. Years ago there were dairies which bottled

milk in amber-colored bottles to protect the milk
from light. The milk was to be kept refrigerated and
sealed except when poured for use. The same prin-
ciples apply to all "living food" after once harvested.
The food should be protected as much as possible
from warmth, light and air."

V.E. Irons, another researcher and an associate of
Dr. C.F. Schnabel (the grass expert), has done much
work in the development of unheated natural supplements from cereal grasses, in a paper (145) entitled
there is a difference he states:

> *"Is it because man believes in Abiogenesis—"the*
> *theory of the production of living from non-living*
> *matter" instead of believing in Biogenesis—"the doc-*
> *trine that living things are produced only from living*
> *things?" Is it because he believes in Natural Science*
> *for things OUTSIDE himself, but for the INNER*
> *MAN he thinks that dead refined foods, dead syn-*
> *thetic vitamins and dead inert materials are as bene-*
> *ficial as live NATURAL FOODS with their live*
> *vitamins and organic minerals, all organized by the*
> *sun, rain, water, minerals, and the soil's living bac-*
> *teria. THERE IS A VAST DIFFERENCE and the*
> *chromatograms show it.*
>
> *"Orthodox Nutrition . . . depends on chemical analy-*
> *sis to determine food values but it is fundamental that*
> *live organic natural foods must be killed (and thus*
> *rendered dead and inert) to be chemically analyzed.*
> *Hence, they may show up as chemically identical to a*
> *synthetic food or vitamin. But the chromatogram*
> *shows the difference.*
>
> *"Many so-called experts still insist that IN-ORGANIC*
> *minerals are as nutritionally effective as the ORGA-*
> *NIZED minerals Nature puts in our foods. If this is*
> *true then why can't we all be readily free of all min-*
> *eral deficiency, because every mineral is available and*
> *very cheap in its inorganic form. However, new evi-*
> *dence indicates that both vitamins and trace minerals,*

to be beneficially effective, must be bound up in Enzyme systems.

"Enzymes are found only in raw, fresh Natural Foods. THERE IS A DIFFERENCE as shown by the chromatograms."

WHAT IS A CHROMATOGRAM

V.E. Irons (145) relates the history of this valuable tool of nutrient analysis:

"The Chromatogram has been used in urine analysis since 1944 but in 1953 Ehrenfried E. Pfeiffer M.D., internationally known soil expert perfected it for graphically demonstrating hidden differences in soils. He knew that frequently two soils might have almost identical chemical analysis but differ widely in biological values such as yield, quality of protein, and seed germination. Its value rests upon the property of certain specially manufactured filter papers, through which individual fractions of a certain substance may be separated, then in turn be made visible by means of a reagent.

The resulting picture allows interpretation through distinct difference in color, rings, spike like forms, etc. as related to qualitative and biological values. These interpretations can be made by anyone who studies them carefully working from a chromatogram of the well known live product to the one under interpretation.

In Nature not only does every living thing have a purpose but its juice displays a definite PATTERN in a chromatogram, whether it be a grain of wheat, a drop of milk, an apple, egg or blade of grass, the fresher the product the greater the biological activity and the more prominent the enzyme formations. But an inorganic mineral, chemical or synthetic vitamin show only varied colored rings but no definite pattern, for they are inert."

116

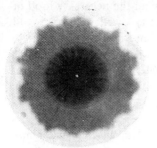

Alpha—tocopherol commercial Vitamin E only a part of complete E complex.

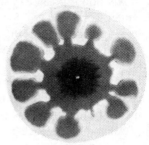

Wheat Germ Oil unheated, which contains Vitamin E complex.

SPROUTING FOR BEGINNERS

For an economical adventure in eating, as an alternative to synthetic foods, try sprouting grains, seeds, legumes or nuts. They can be grown simply in any container with daily watering. For the more serious adventurer, ½ in. of soil or few sheets of paper towels will simulate a garden indoors to provide you an abundant harvest in 3 to 8 days. It requires minimal space, for example, ¼ cup lentils (or mung) will fill a quart size jar with sprouts in 4 days. Or if you grow a half pound of sunflower seeds (birdfood) on a typical baker tray (18 x 24 in.) you will produce about four pounds of delicious salad greens that taste slightly like watercress, use it in salads, on sandwiches, in casseroles, juice it.

The cost of these organic greens is about 5¢ per pound. During the winter months in most cities, you can expect to pay at least ten times that for food that is nutritionally inferior. These seeds when stored will provide high nutritional food to your family if the city should become paralyzed by a strike, riot, fuel shortage, or crop failure.

An indoor green can supply all the necessary food in winter (or summer) for the city dweller. Sprouts and immature greens are the most nutritious and live, raw, organic food that is available on this planet. They are still growing at the dinner table. Hence, no nutritional loss due to time lapse between harvest and serving. This can be significant; for instance, a 5 day delay in shipment of oranges means a 50% loss of vitamin C.

Although raw food is best, those who are not ready for a complete live food diet, may add raw sprouts to all cooked dishes just before serving. Even this slight gesture will reward you with improved health.

Dried legumes cook faster if they are sprouted. They also provide more bulk and nutrition without increased cost. This reduction in cooking time will minimize air pollution and help to conserve fuel. Furthermore, sprouting eliminates the aftereffects of stomach gas which is associated with cooked beans.

Isn't It Time You Fell In Love With A Sprout

Sprouts and indoor greens make a perfect vitamin-rich substitute for fruits and vegetables. They also provide you with a complete balanced protein in a pre-digested form which is easily and efficiently assimilated by your body. The vitamins and enzyme activity is at its peak, never to be surpassed as the "anti-cancer vitamin" increases a hundred times over its initial value in seed because of sprouting. The "virility vitamin" E triples in four days in wheat through sprouting. The starch and fat is converted to sugar and carbohydrates providing you with quick high energy.

You can grow your own organic greens in portable gardens. They can be grown in any room, or any make of car, even in your backpack or tuxedo jacket pocket.

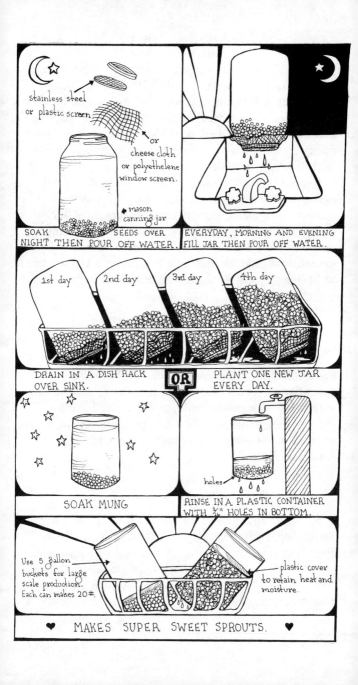

Sprouts Are Coming

For equipment, the simplest method is to get a large mouth quart size, or larger, glass jar. A small piece of nylon net, or polyethelene window screen can be obtained from a local hardware store. You can also use cheese cloth or strainer. A rubber band or a jar rim, the kind that is found on canning jars, will hold cheese-cloth or screen in place.

Select sprouting quality seeds—be sure they are not old or treated with chemicals. Some authorities recommend using mold inhibitors in sprouting, this is completely unnecessary if you have quality seeds and follow instructions. Purchase seeds that have at least 88% germination ratio, i.e. out of 100 seeds you can be sure of having at least 88 seeds which will sprout perfectly.

I Was Munged By A Sprout

Easiest to sprout are the mung and alfalfa seeds which can be purchased at most health food stores. Lentils are the easiest seeds to locate. They can be found in any supermarket. Lentils are good seeds to try for the first experience in sprouting. In one quart size jar place ¼ cup of lentil or mung, or 2 tablespoons of alfalfa, or a mixture of 3 tablespoons of mung, and 1 tablespoon of lentil and alfalfa.

Would Rather Sprout Than Switch

Remove any broken or cracked seeds. Wash the seeds thoroughly. Put the seeds back in a jar. Cover it with lukewarm (not from hot water faucet) water, make sure it is at least twice the volume of the seeds. If available use distilled or spring water. Ann Wigmore has observed that few dozen blades of grass immersed in the water for the soaking period, will counteract the

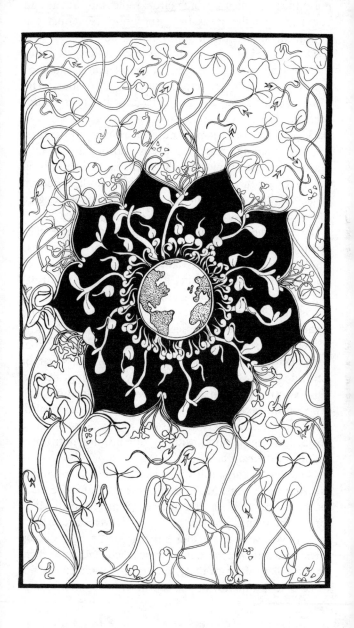

poisonous chemicals which are in the tap water and could prevent the seeds from sprouting. Next, place a net on jar and secure it with band or cover.

During soaking the seeds will swell to several times their original size. Soak alfalfa about 4 hours, mung or lentils about 16 hours, and mixture 12 to 16 hours. The exact soaking times are not very critical. During summer one can cut down the soaking time. Keep seeds in dark place at room temperature of at least 70 degrees.

After soaking, rinse the seeds thoroughly in luke warm water and drain well. Keep the screen and lid on jar. Place jar in any bowl, with a folded cloth in bottom to absorb the water. Tilt the jar to about a 45 degree angle, open end down, keep in a dark warm space.

Except when taken out for rinsing, the sprouting seeds should remain in the dark cupboard. Thoroughly rinse and drain at least twice daily. After about 3 days of sprouting one discovers that if one misses a day of rinsing there will be no damage done to the sprouts. If the air is very hot or dry, give the seeds longer and more frequent rinses, use cold or iced water.

When the seeds start to sprout, hulls will separate from seed. During rinsing, they have a tendency to float or settle to the bottom. By temporarily removing the net, the loose mung or alfalfa hulls may be scooped off with a spoon or the alfalfa hulls rinsed away. The removal of hulls is not absolutely necessary, but it does improve taste and digestibility, without diminishing nutritional value. Furthermore, it reduces sprout spoilages.

The day to eat sprouts is personal and will be guided by your taste buds. Most people prefer alfalfa when it is at least 6 days old and the two leaves are formed. Many prefer the mungs just before the two leaves start appearing. If you soak the mung initially for 24 hours, keep them in a very warm, damp, dark place, and rinse them at least 4 to 6 times daily, letting the water run for at least 3 to 5 minutes at warm temperature. After about

2 to 3 days one will get very sweet tasty sprouts—just like fresh peas. If allowed to grow for 4 days under these conditions, then one gets a total conversion of starch into sugar and they make excellent vegetables for juicing. Lentils, when used for salad are at their best in 2 days, but for juicing allow them to grow for at least 5 days.

Stop Being R.I.P.ped Off, Heal With Mother Nature

When the small leaves are formed, you might want to develop chlorophyll. This can be done by placing the jar near a window for 2 to 8 hours for the absorption of indirect sunlight. The green blood of the plant is the regenerator of the human temple. Be sure your sprouts have some of it. Don't allow sprouts to overheat and spoil because of placing sprout on a metallic surface.

I Was Reborn On Sprouts

When you are ready to harvest the sprouts, give them the final rinse—try to remove the remaining hulls—then drain and store in the refrigerator. Keep them in a plastic bag or glass jar. They will remain fresh and continue to grow slowly in the refrigerator for up to several weeks. Before serving them, it is always a good nutritional practice to rinse them and expose them to indirect sunlight for at least two hours.

Before starting the next batch, wash the strainer and jar in hot water to prevent mold or fungus from forming.

Sprouts Make Such Nice Roommates

Other excellent seeds for sprouting are fenugreek, wheat, rye, soy, radish, unhulled or hulled—uncracked sunflower, peanuts, almonds. The average soaking time is 12 hours.

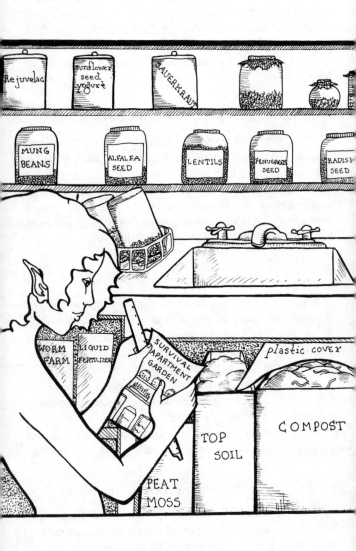

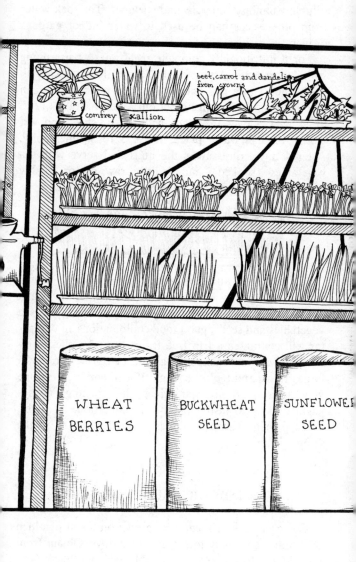

The soak water of alfalfa, fenugreek, and grains can be used as a drink. It will provide a rich source of water soluble vitamins, minerals, and enzymes. The soak water from other seeds can be used to water indoor gardens or plants.

For a nutritionally complete meal mix 6 parts mung with 1 part lentil, 1 part alfalfa, 1 part fenugreek. Soak for 12 hours in a jar. Then sprout this mixture in a can or bucket which has in its bottom a dozen holes (1/16 to 1/8 in.). Cover the seeds with plastic sheet and wet cloth. Keep in warm place. Rinse 3 to 5 times daily. After 4 days, rinse away the hulls and serve with sea vegetables (soaked) and a little raw oil or freshly ground sunflower or sesame seeds or seed yogurt.

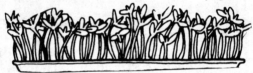

For those of you who are travelling by car, you will find sprouting very easy in wide mouth quart size jars. Add to your lunchbasket fruit, fresh and dried, plus sea vegetables and seeds, good food combinations and laughter will guarantee a trip free from stomach aches. Similarly, if you are backpacking, you can grow sprouts in large, transparent plastic bags. Use them in the same way as a quart size jar. Keep the openings always slightly loose to insure plenty of ventilation. At night, to keep them warm, take them to bed with you in the sleeping bag.

INDOOR GARDENING

Generally indoor greens are grown on about one inch of soil and are ready to eat in 5 to 9 days. Obtain from the natural foods store sproutable wheat; "black, un-

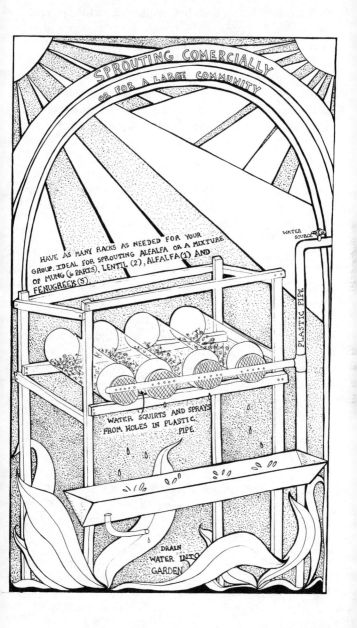

SPROUTING COMERCIALLY

or for a large community

HAVE AS MANY RACKS AS NEEDED FOR YOUR GROUP. IDEAL FOR SPROUTING ALFALFA OR A MIXTURE OF MUNG (6 PARTS), LENTIL (2), ALFALFA (1) AND FENUGREEK (5).

WATER SOURCE

PLASTIC PIPE

WATER SQUIRTS AND SPRAYS FROM HOLES IN PLASTIC PIPE.

DRAIN WATER INTO GARDEN.

hulled buckwheat"; unhulled sunflower; radish; or fenugreek. Soak the wheat 15 hours, the buckwheat about 4 hours, and the others at least 10 hours.

Fill a baking pan (or any other flat tray) with dark, porous, pleasant smelling soil. Fifty percent peat moss (purchased from a green house or garden supply center) will make the soil more porous. Mix in 1 tablespoon of kelp fertilizer (optional). Moisten the soil—no puddles. Spread the seed next to one another. Cover loosely with a plastic sheet or a little soil. Put in a wam dark place. After 3 days remove the cover. Place the tray in a light area. Water as neded. After four or more additional days it is ready to harvest—an economical source of sun vibrations during the cold winter.

You Live A Little Longer On Grass

After the harvest, wheat can be allowed to regrow for two additional times. The other seeds sometimes will produce a second harvest. The mats of earth and stubs can be accumulated and when worms and bacteria are allowed to act on it, you can expect total decomposition of the soil into earth which can be used again in planting. This generally takes at least 8 weeks. Keep the earth in barrels with holes in them. Water as needed.

When the use of soil and composting seems to be impractical, the following methods of growing can be considered:

a.) The soil may be replaced with 4 layers of wet paper towel, or one layer of white cotton or linen towel. It is very important to keep the towels moist and the pan in a warm place, especially during the first three days.

b.) Instead of trays, use a 12 inch plastic or steel screen placed in a wood frame. It can be purchased in a hardware store as window screen. Over the screen

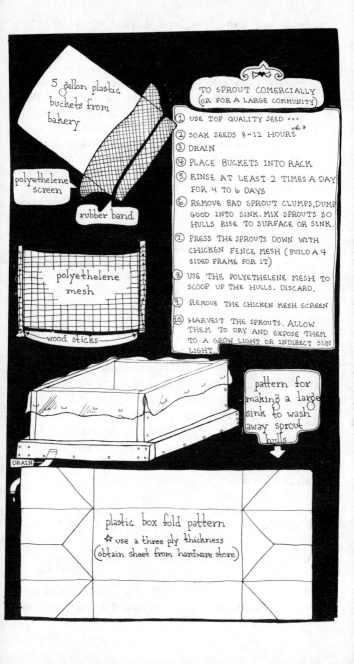

place wet white linen or cheesecloth. Cover densely, as in planting on soil, with soaked wheat seeds (or any other seeds). Cover the wheat with at least 1 layer of damp cloth. You can build a rack to hold at least 4 frames. Daily take rack to sink and mist gently with warm water. After draining return rack to place. The top cover should be removed by fourth day.

c.) A half cup of wheat (sunflower, fenugreek, radish) can be sprouted to a grass in a wide mouth quart size jar (or even a strainer). After 3 days of sprouting, for better ventilation, tip bottle on side. Be sure to keep the water thoroughly drained.

d.) Soil may be replaced with peat moss. Purchase kelp liquid seaweed fertilizer. Follow instructions for preparing a solution. Mix into peat moss. Should feel thoroughly moist without pockets of water. Press this peat moss mixture into a tray, just as you would be preparing a pie crust, about 1/4 to 3/8 inch thick. Plant the seeds. Water as needed daily.

WHEATGRASS: Chew on the grass, sucking in the juice, spitting out the pulp. If you have a special juicer you may extract ten ounces of juice from one pound of grass (this requires about ¼ pound of wheat seeds). You might want to use a meat grinder or a grain mill on the grass. Take the finely ground pulp and press it through a strainer or squeeze it through a cheese cloth to get the juice out. The grass may be cut very fine, especially when it is less than 4 days old, and added to salads or blended with other foods. It should be added to all cooked foods just before serving.

Do You Want To Live . . . Grass Has More To Give

Wheatgrass (as well as other grasses) is a complete food and is very rich in chlorophyll—a good body builder with its easily assimilable protein. Daily, at least one ounce should be taken as a survival cocktail for those

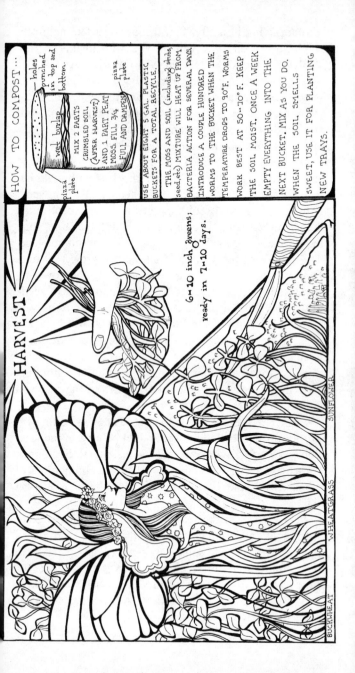

HOW TO COMPOST...

MIX 2 PARTS CRUMBLED SOIL (AFTER HARVEST) AND 1 PART PEAT MOSS. FILL 3/4 FULL AND DAMPEN.

holes punched in top and bottom.

wet burlap

pizza plate

USE ABOUT EIGHT 5 GAL. PLASTIC BUCKETS FOR A TOTAL RECYCLE.

THE MOSS AND SOIL (including scraps, seed, etc) MIXTURE WILL HEAT UP FROM BACTERIA ACTION FOR SEVERAL DAYS. INTRODUCE A COUPLE HUNDRED WORMS TO THE BUCKET WHEN THE TEMPERATURE DROPS TO 90°F. WORMS WORK BEST AT 50~70°F. KEEP THE SOIL MOIST. ONCE A WEEK EMPTY EVERYTHING INTO THE NEXT BUCKET. MIX AS YOU DO. WHEN THE SOIL SMELLS SWEET, USE IT FOR PLANTING NEW TRAYS.

HARVEST

6~10 inch greens; ready in 7~10 days.

BUCKWHEAT

WHEATGRASS

SUNFLOWER

who are living in a city. It will make you feel naturally "high" every day and will fill you with loving energy.

BUCKWHEAT AND SUNFLOWER: After it is fully grown, remove any remaining husks and use as salad green or juice it. Rich in amino acids, enzymes, vitamins, chlorophyll, low in fat, free from starch. Both are good sources of vitamin D and lecithin. Slightly salty. Much more palatable than wheatgrass.

On maturity, in about 8 days, one can harvest the entire crop by cutting close to the soil with a knife. Refrigerate in plastic bag. It will keep well for a week. If the temperature is cold, the greens can be kept much longer on the soil. If refrigeration is not available, time the vegetation growth so that there will be no spoilage. The sunflower turns bitter if allowed to grow too long. However, the buckwheat is delicious up to the flowering stage. It is a good practice to plant enough extra seeds in the real outdoor soil so that you will be able to harvest a crop of sunflower and buckwheat which will be available for the sprouting. Buckwheat makes a very delicious juice as it gets older.

Since the seeds have an uneven rate of sprouting, after the harvest, you will notice that from the mat you can expect a second crop from the slow starters.

FENUGREEK AND RADISH: Tangy seasoning for exotic sprout salad additions. Should be used in moderation. Powerful liver and kidney cleansers. Fenugreek tea is especially very useful to speed elimination of mucus from your body. May be sprouted or grown on soil.

POTTING: In the fall, pot at least one dozen comfrey roots (also dandelion) in tall tin cans. Drop in a few earthworms, add some kelp fertilizer and place them in a sunny window. Water as needed with soak (or rinse) water from your sprouts. The 6 to 10 inch leaves may be harvested continuously. A new crop can be expected every two weeks.

Comfrey is valuable nutritionally, as well as noted for its medicinal qualities. Use the leaves for salads, sauces, tea, or steam them lightly. It is a laxative, may be used as a poltice for wounds and chest ailments; hot comfrey tea may be drunk at bedtime to induce sweating.

Blend comfrey leaves with water or carrot juice. Obtain comfrey juice by pouring mixture through a fine strainer or into centrifugal juicer. Or run comfrey leaves, followed by carrot, celery, zuchini, cucumber or beet in a centrifugal juicer. Keep feeding comfrey then carrot in the juicing process.

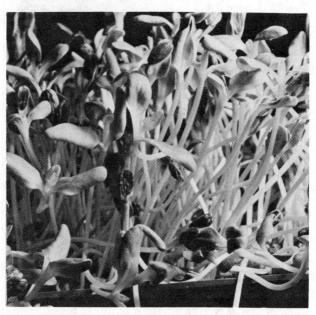

4 day old Sunflower greens grown on ½ inch soil.

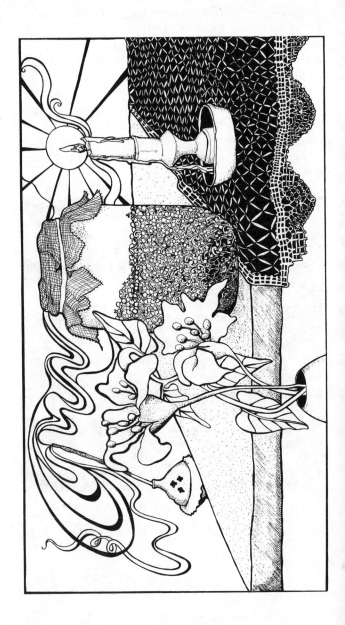

BIBLIOGRAPHY

1. *SZEKELY, E.B., The Essene Gospel of John.* Published by Academy Books, 3085 Reynard Way, San Diego, Cal.

2. *FRENCH, C.E., BERRYMAN, G.H., GOORLEY, J.T., H.A. HARPER, D.M. HARKNESS and E.J. THACHER. "The production of vitamins in germinated peas, soybeans, and other beans."*

3. *MAYER, A.M. and A. POLJAKOFF-MAYBER. The Germination of Seeds.* Pergamon Press, Headington Hill Hall, Oxford, Britain. 1966.

4. *EDITOR. "B vitamins in sprouted cereal grains"* Nutrition Reviews. No. 15. Page 356. October 1943.

5. *AMERICAN MEDICAL ASSOCIATION MONOGRAPH, THE VITAMINS.* 1939. Found in most large medical libraries.

6. *ROSENBERG, H.R. Chemistry and Physiology of the Vitamins.* 1942. Found in Harvard Medical Library, or any large size library.

7. *HLYNKA. WHEAT: CHEMISTRY AND TECHNOLOGY.* Publ. American Association of Cereal Chemists.

8. *NIPPON NOGEI KAGAKU KAISHI. Qualitative distribution of free sugar in organs of various cereals and legumes during germination.* 41:646, 1967.

9. *AGRICULTURE RESEARCH SERVICE, UNITED STATES DEPARTMENT OF AGRICULTURE. Agriculture Handbook No. 1.* Composition of Foods. 1963. Pub. USDA, Wash. D.C.

10. *KUPPUSWAMY, S. PROTEINS IN FOOD. Indian Council of Medical Research, New Delhi,* 1958. Pages 35-39, 46, 229 and 230.

11. *YOUNG J.L. and J.E. VARNER. Arch Biochem Biophys* 84:71, 1959.

12. *HARDMAN, E.E. and W.M. CROMBIE, J. Exp Bot.* 9:239, 1958.

13. *BOATMAN, S.G. and W.M. CROMBIE, J. Exp Bot.* 9:52, 1958.

14. *YAMADA, M. Sc Paper Coll Gen Ed Univer Tokyo.* 5:161, 1955.

15. *ORR M.L. and B.K. WATT. Amino Acid Content of Foods.* Home Economics Research Report No. 4 U.S. Government Printing Office, Washington, D.C.

16. *VIRTANEN, A.I., A.M. BERG and S. KARI. ACTA Chem Scand.* 7:1423, 1953.

17. *BURKHOLDER, P.R. and I. McVEIGH, Increase of B. Vitamins in Germinating Seeds Proc.* N.A.S. 28:440, 1942.

18. *CHATTOPADHYAY, H. and S. BANERJEE, Studies on the ascorbic acid oxidase activity of some common Indian pulses during germination.* Ind. Jour. Med. Res. 40:439, 1952.

19. *CHATTOPADHYAY, H. and S. BANERJEE. Studies on the clorine content of some common Indian pulses and cereals both before an during the course of germination.* Food Res. 16:230, 1951.

20. *BANERJEE, SATCHITANANDA, MAYA BANERJEE and KRISHNASUDHA ROHATGI, "Effect of Germination on the total Tocopherol Content of Pulses and Cereal,"* Journal of Food Science, 17:402-3, 1952.

21. *CHATTOPADHYAY, H. and S. BANERJEE. Effect of germination on the carotene content of pulses and cereals.* Science 113:600, 1951.

22. *NAUTILUS MAGAZINE, quoted by R. Colliers, Law of the Higher Potential.* Collier Publishers, Tarrytown, New York, 1947, p. 232.

23. *PRICE, W.A. Nutritional and Physical Regeneration,* Lee Foundation of Physical Research, Milwaukee, Wisconsin, 1945.

24. *ROHATGI, K., BANERJEE M. and S. BANERJEE. Effect of germination on vitamin B12 values of pulses.* Jour. Nutrition 56:403-408, 1955.

25. *ALTMAN, P. and D. DITTMAN. Metabolism.* Federation of America Society for Experimental Biology. Publ.

26. *ELLWOOD, C. Feel like a Million.* Pocket Books, 1 West 39th St., New York, New York, 75§, 1969.

27. *BURKHOLDER, P.R. Vitamins in dehydrated seeds and sprouts.* Science, 97:562, 1943.

28. *HERTING, D.C., J.E. EMMA, Alpha tocopherol content of cereal grains and processed cereals.* Agri. Food Chem. 17:785, 1969.

29. *LINKO AND MILNER, Cereal Chem.* 36:280, 1959.

30. *KOZMINA, and ROMANOVA, Biochem.* 3:378, 1938.

31. *LEE, J.Y., C.Y. LEE, T.Y. LEE, T.W. KNON. Chemical Changes during germination of soybeans: carbohydrate metabolism.* Seoul Univ. J. 9:12, 1959.

32. *WAI, TSO, BISHOP, MACK, COTTON. Plant Physiology.* 22:117, 1947.

33. *KIRSCHNER, H.E. Nature's Healing Grasses.* H.C. White Publications, P.O. Box 8014, Riverside, California 92501. Price $2.00.

34. *GUGGOLOZ, J. V.V. HERRING and G. O. KOHLER, Dehydrated Alfalfa Composition. Correlation of nutrient components with Protein content.* Agriculture and Food Chemistry. 15:1052, 1967.

35. *BINGER, H.P., C.R. THOMPSON and G.O. KOHLER. Composition of Dehydrated forages, Technical Bulletin No. 1235.* Issued January 1961. Superintendent of Documents, U.S. Government Printing Office, Washington 25, D.C.

36. *BIOCHEM J.* 1968, 108, p. 468.

37. *BURKHOLDER and McVEIGH:* Proc N.A.S. ol. 28, 1942, pg. 440.

38. *LEOHR, FRANKLIN, "The Power of Prayer"* on plants.

39. *SAUNDERS C. W. Proc. Soc. Exp. Bible, N.Y.,* 23:788, 1925.

40. *EVANS & BUTTS,* Science 190: 569, 1949.

41. *OLSEN, Canadian T of Biochem.,* 45:1673, 1967.

42. *YOCUM L. E., J. AGROM,* Res. 31, 727, 1925.

43. *SEMENKO G.I., FIZIOL.* Rusteny 4, 332, 1957.

44. *CANCER NEWS JOURNAL,* Aug. 1970. (C.C.S., 2043 N. Berendo, L.A., Cal.)

45. *NEWSWEEK,* July 9, 1973, p. 69.

46. *VOISIN, ANDRE, "Soil Grass and Cancer",* Crosby, Lockwood & Son Ltd., 26 Old Brompton Rd., SW 7, London 1959.

47. *NATURAMA HEALTH CARE,* Hippocrates Health Institute, 25 Exeter St., Boston, Mass.

48. *WIGMORE, ANN. Be Your Own Doctor,* H.H.I., 25 Exeter St., Boston, Mass.

49. *KULVINSKAS V., Survival into 21st Century.* OMango d'Press, P.O. Box 255, Wethersfield, Conn.

50. *LOEHR, F., The Power of Prayer on Plants* (The New American Library Inc., Bergenfield, N.J.)

51. *BOSTON SUNDAY ADVERTISER,* May p. 7, 1970, Section, 2A, page 1.

52. *KOHLER, G.O., C.A. ELVEHJEM and E.B. HART; Growth Stimulating properties of grass juice.* Science, 83:445, 1936.

53. *KOHLER, G.O., C.A. ELVEHJEM and E.B. HART; Further studies on the growth promoting factor associated with summer milk.* J. Nutr. 14:131, 1937.

54. *KOHLER, G.O.C.A. ELVEHJEM, and E.B. HART, The relation of the 'grass juice factor' to guinea pigs nutrition.* J. Nutr. 15:445, 1938.

55. *KOHLER, G.O. Unidentified Factors Relating Reproduction in animals Feedstuffs,* August 8, 1953.

56. *VIRTANEN, A.I. Vitamins and plants,* Nature, 137:779, 1936.

57. *VIRTANEN, A.I. and T. LAINE, Amino acids of plants at different stages of growth.* Nature, 137;237, 1936a.

58. *ALTMAN, P. and D. DITTMER, Metabolism,* Published by American Society for Experimental Biology. Bethesda, Maryland.

59. *AGRICULTURE RESEARCH SERVICE, United States Department of Agriculture.* Agriculture Handbook No. 8 Composition of Foods.

60. *HUNT, C.H., P.R. RECORD and R.M. BETHKE, The influence of the stage of maturity on the chemical composition and vitamin B (b1) and G content of hays and pasture grasses.* Ohio Agr. Exp. Sta. Bull. 576, 1936.

61. *PFEIFFER, E.E. Protein changes during germina-*

tion and earliest leaf growth. Bio-Dynamics, 47:2, 1958, R.D. 1. Chester, N.Y.

62. *FREE PRESS WEEKLY,* page 9 Dec. 14, 1968, Western Canada.

63. *ABDERHALDEN, E. LEHRBUCH DER PHYSIOLOGISHEN CHEMIE IN DREISSIG VORLESUNGEN,* ed. 3, Berlin, Urban & Schwarcenberg, 1914.

64. *VERDEIL, M.F. COMPT,* rend. Acad. d. sc., 33:689, 1851.

65. *HOPPE-SEYLER, F. ZTSCHR.* f. physiol. Chem. 3: 339, 1879; 4:193, 1880.

66. *WILLSTATTER, R. and STOLLK. Unterschungen ueber Chlorophyll,* Berlin, Julius Springer, 1913.

67. *WILLSTATER AND ASCHINA. Oxydation der Chlorophyll Derivative.* Ann., 373, :227, 1910, Uber die Reduction des Chlorophyll. ibid., 385:188, 1911.

68. *FISHER, Nobelvortrag Stockholm 1931,* Z. Angew, Chemie, 44:617, 1931.

69. *EDITOR. Determination and quantitative estimation of the decomposition of chlorophyll in the human body.* Staff Meetings of the Mayo Clinic. 13:95, 1938.

70. *FOWLER, E.P. PLACEBOS,* anti-sludging drugs and disorders of the ear. Ann Otol. 70:839, 1961.

71. *SMITH, L.W. Remarks upon the history, chemistry, toxicity and antibacterial properties of watersoluble chlorophyll derivatives as therapeutic agents.* Am J. of the Med. Science. 207:649, 1944.

72. *WOLF. Influence of the day length on the chlorophyll content of wheat seedling.* Phy. Rev. Int. Bot. Exp 21:01, 1964.

73. *BURGI, E. Cor.-Bl. F. Schweiz. Aerzte,* 46:449, 1916.

74. *SCOTT, E. and C.J. DELOR.* Ohio State M.J. 29:165, 1933.

75. *SCOTT, J.M.D. Biochem J.* 17:157, 1923.

76. *PATEK, A.J. Chlorophyll and regeneration of the blood.* Archives of Internal Medicine, 47:76, 1936.

77. *SAUNDERS, C.W. Proc. Soc. exp. Biol. N.Y.* 23:788, 1925.

78. *PATEK and MINOT, "Bile pigment and hemo-*

globin regeneration. The effect of bile pigment in cases of chronic hyperchromic anemia," Am J. Med. Science. 188:206, 1934.

79. *MILLER, L.M.* "Chlorophyll for healing." Sc News Letter, March 15 1941, p. 171.

80. *BINET, I. and M.W. STRUMZA,* Sang, 8:1041, 1934.

81. *LOUROU, M. and O. LARTIGUE.* "The influence of diet on the biological effects produced by whole body irradiation." Experientai. 6:25, 1950.

82. *BURGI, E. and C. F. VON TRACZEWSHY,* Biochem. Z., 98:256, 1919.

83. *AOKI, S. SEI-KWAI Med. J.,* 50:1, 1931, Chem. Abst. 26;3847, 1932.

84. *ZICHGRAF, G/Munch.* Med. Woch., 79:998, 1932.

85. *ROTHEMUND, P. R. MCNARY and O.L. INMAN,* J. Am. Chem. Soc. 56:2400, 1934.

86. *HUGHES, J.H. and A.L. LATNER* "Chlorophyll and hemoglobin regeneration after hemorrhage." J. Physiology, 86:388, 1936.

87. *ZIH, A. Pfugers Arch.* 225:728, 1930.

88. *SPOEHR, H.A.* "The chemical aspects of photosynthesis". Stanford Annual Review of Biochemistry, 2:453, 1936.

89. *DIETZ, E.M.* "Chlorophyll and Hemoglobin-two natural pyrrole pigments". J Chem Educ. May 1935, p. 208.

90. *BURGI, E.* Das Chlorophyll Als Pharmakon, Leipzig, Georg Thieme, 1932.

91. *BOWERS, W.S.* "Chlorophyll in wound healing and suppurative disease." Am. J. Surg. 73:37, 1947.

92. *MORGAN, W.S.:* The Therapeutic use of Chlorophyll. Gutherie Clin. Bull. 16:94, 1947.

93. *BOEHME, E.J.:* The Treatment of Chronic Leg Ulcers with Special Reference to ointment containing water-soluble Chlorophyll. Lahey Clin. Bull. 4:242, 1946.

94. *SMITH, L.W. and A.E. LIVINGSTON.* "Chlorophyll: An experimental study of its water-soluble derivatives in wound healing." Am. J. Surg. 52:358, 1943.

95. *BERTRAM, R.O. and B.S. WEINSTOCK.* "A

*clinical evaluation of chlorophyll, Benzocaine and urea
ointment in treatment of minor infections of the foot."* J.
Am. Podiat Assoc. 19:366, 1959.

96. *GRUSKIN, B.* Amer. J. Surgery, 49:49, 1940.

97. *OFFENKRANTZ, W.G. "Water Soluble chlorophyll in the treatment of peptic ulcers of long duration."*
Rev. Gastroenterology, 17:359, 1950.

98. *CARPENTER, E.B. "Clinical experiences with
chlorophyll preparations with particular reference to chronic
osteomyelitis and chronic ulcer".* Am. J. Surgery. 77:167,
1949.

99. *JUUL-MOLLER and A.V. MIKKELSEN. "Treatment of hypertension and crural ulcer with chlorophyllin"*
Ugesk. laeger. 114:1726, 1952.

100. *CARLESEN, R. and P. GARSYEN. "Septofyllin
(chlorophyll preparation) especially in chronic leg ulcer".*
Nord. Med. 47:412, 1952.

101. *RAFSKY H.A. and C.I. KRIEGER. "Treatments
of intestinal diseases with solutions of water-solluble
chlorophyll"* Rev. Gastroenterology. 15:549, 1948.

102. *PALOSCIA, F. and G. PALLOTTEN. "Chlorophyll therapy."* Lotta. Contra. Tuberc. 22:738, 1952.

103. *"RESULTS OF CHLOROPHYLL THERAPY."*
Bull Assoc. Franc Pol'etude du Cancer. 24:15. 1935.

104. *PLAGNIEL "Remarkable tonic power of chlorophyll pigment in asthenic toxemia of Cancer."* J. de. med.
de. Paris. 53:664, 1933.

105. *"Chlorophyll therapy for Cancer."* Progress. Med.
Ap 6, 1935, pg. 583.

106. *DUPLAN, J.F. "Influence of dietary regimen on
radiosensitivity of the guinea pig."* Compt. rend, acad. sci.
236:424, 1953.

107. *SPECTOR, H. and D. H. CALLOWAY, "Reduction of X-radiation mortality by cabbage and broccoli".*
Proc. Soc. Exptl. Biol. Med. 100:405, 1959.

108. *COLLOWAY, D.H., W.K. CALHOUN and A. H.
Munson "Further studies on reduction of X-irradiation
mortality of guinea pigs by plant materials."* Quartermaster
Food and Container Institute for the Armed Forces
Report NR. 12-61, 1961.

109. *AMMANN, E.C.B. and V.H. LYNCH*, "Purine metabolism by unicellular alegy 111. The photochemical degradation of uric acid by chlorophyll". Biochemica et Biophysica ACTA. 120:181, 1966.

110. *MILLER, J.M., D.A. JACKSON and C.S. COLLIER*, "The institution of clotting by chlorophyllin." Am. J. Surgery. 95: 967, 1958.

111. *THOMPKINS, P. and BIRD, C. The Secret Life of Plants*. Avon Books, N.Y.C. 1973.

112. *FLANAGAN, C.P.* Ph. D. Pyramid Power, Pyramid Publishers, 438 W. Cypress St. Glendale, Ca.

113. *THE NATUROPATH*, Sep. 1969. (1920 N. Kilpatrick St., Portland, Oregon)

114. *VOISSIN*, Trail Diary, U.S.A. Mission Forage Production, Vol. 11, p. 379.

115. *ACRES, U.S.A.* (March, April, May, July, August) 1973. Box 1456, Kansas City, Mo.

116. *V.E. IRONS* (11S Main St., Natick, Mass.)

117. *HOTEMA, Hilton*. Man's Higher Consciousness. Health Research, Mokelumne Hill, Cal.

118. *CURTIS, C. An Account of the Disease of India as they appeared in the English Fleet*. Edinburg 1807.

TOBE J.H. 1970 Sprouts, Elixir Of Life. St. Catharines, Ontario, Canada: Provoker Press.

OLIVER, H.O., 1975, Add a few Sprouts, Keats Publ. Inc., New Canaan, Conn.

119. *NORDFELDT, S.* Effect of germination upon total tocopherols in wheat. K. Lantbrukshogskolans Ann. 28:181-188; 1962.

120. *LISLE, HARVEY* (RD 1, Norwalk, Ohio)

121. *RADHAKRISHNAN A.N.; VAIDYANATHAN C.S. and K.V. GIRI, Nitrogenous constituents in plants.* I Free Amino Acids in leaves and leguminous seeds. Tour. Ind. Inst. Sci. 37:178-194, 1957.

122. *EMBREY h. and T.C. WANG Analyses of some Chinese Foods*. China Med. Jour. 35:247-257, 1921.

123. *NANDI, D.S. Studies on the changes in free amino acids and B-vitamin content of some leguminous seeds during germination*. Sci and Cult. 23:659-660, 1958.

124. *BROWN B.E., MEADE, E.M. and J.R. BUTTER-*

FIELD. *The effect of germination upon the fact of soybean.* Jour. Am. Oil Chem. Soc. 39: 327-330; 1962.

125. *WHITE H.B. Jr., Fat utilization and composition in germinated cotton seeds.* Plant physiol. 33:218, 1958.

126. *PFEIFFER, E.C. Protein changes during germination and earliest leaf growth.* Bio-Dynamics, 47:2, 1958 (Bio-Dynamic Farms, R.D. 1, Chester, N.Y.)

127. *ENCYCLOPEDIA BRITTANICA,* 30 volumes, Macropaedia Vol. 16, "Knowledge in Depth", Founded 1768, 15th Ed. 1974.

128. *MELLANBY, EDWARD, Journal of Physiology,* 109:488-533, 1949. Experimental animals. London.

129. *FRY E., ALLRED J., JENSEN L., and J. MCGINNIS, Department of Poultry Science, State College of Washington.* Influence of water treatment on nutritional value of barley. Proceedings of the society for Experimental Biology and Medicine. 95:249-251, 1951.

130. *MCELROY, W.P. Director of the McCullom Pratt Institute,* John Hopkins University before Nat. Academy of Science, Wash., D.C.

131. *DUNCAN, GARFIELD, G., M.D., Diseases of Metabolism.* 3rd edition. Includes article by T. Spies, M.D.

132. *BICKNELL AND PRESCOTT,* Vitamins in *Medicine.* p. 688. 1946.

133. *MORGAN, A.F., Science,* March 14, 1941.

134. *JOURNAL OF THE A.M.A.* 126:437, 1944.

135. *POTTENGER, F.M. Oral Surgery,* 32:8, 467-485, Aug. 1946. And, What is New in Farm Science, U-Wisc., Nov. 1938, p. 84.

136. *PROCEEDINGS OF THE NUTRITIONAL SOCIETY,* Seventy first scientific meeting, London School of Hygiene and Tropical medicine, Jan. 5, 1952. Vitamin B-12, page 295.

137. *BENERJEE, D.K. and J.B. CHATTERJEA. Vitamin B-12 content of some articles of Indian diet and effect of cooking on it.* Bri. J. Nutr. 17:385, 1963.

138. *ZICHGRAF, G.* Munch. Wed. Wach. 79:998, 1932 and SAUNDERS, C.W., Pro. Soc. Exp. Biol. N.Y. 23:788, 1925.

139. *FRANK, BENJAMIN S., M.D., Nucleic Acid*

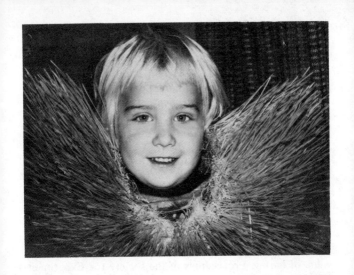

Therapy in Aging and Degenerative disease, Psychological Library Publishers, NYC.

140. *MAROTI M*. Acta Biologica Academiae, Scientiarum Hungaricae VII, 277, 1957.

141. *SEMENKO, G.I.*, Fiziol. Rasteny 4:332, 1957.

142. *ROBERTS, D.W.A.*, J. Biochem. Physiol. 39:-1333, 1961

143. *LEAF, A., M.D., Every Day is a Gift When You are over 100.* National Geographic 143:1, 93-119, 1973.

144. *WIGMORE, ANN, Spiritual Diet*, Hippocrates Health Institute, 25 Exeter St., Boston, Mass.

145. *IRONS, V.E., There is a Difference*, V.E. Irons Inc., 11S. Main St. Natick, Mass.

146. *KAKADE, M.L. and R.J. EVANS*, Journal of Food Science, 31:781, 1966.

147. *HEGAZI, S.M.*, Zeitschrift fur Ernahrungswissenschraft, 13:200, 1974.

148. *McLEOD, TRAVIS, WREY*, J. Inst. Brew., 59: 154, 1953.

149. *BURR, G.O., BURR, M.M., J. BIOL. CHE.*, 82: 345, 1929; 86:587, 1930.

150. J. Sci. Food and Agri., 9:505, 1958.

151. *SHERMAN H.C.*, J. of Franklin Inst. 125th. Aniv. No., p. 95, Jan. 1951.

SEED AND OTHER RESOURCES

JUICE SUITE, P.O. Box 701, Bloomfield, CT 06002 Grass juicers distillers, blenders and vegetable juicers. Discount on many of the appliances. Send 50¢ for literature.

HELTON DIST., 2741 Sequoia, Fullerton, Ca. 92634. Large variety sold in one pound quantities.

CHAMPLAIN VALLEY SEED, Box 454, Westport, New York 12993. Buckwheat.

MEER CORP., Mallincott, New York, (212) 586-0900. Fenugreek, $200 minimal.

DIAMOND K ENTERPRISES St. Charles, MN 55972 932-4308. Sunflower seed. Request black ones used in oil making.

LIVING FARMS, 200 3rd St., Tracy, Minnesota, 56175. Alfalfa, wheat, rye, and red clover.

CROSS SEED CO., Route 1, Box 125, Bunker Hill, Kansas 67676. Alfalfa, wheat, rye.

G. CRANE, Creek Road, Craftsbury, Vt. 05826. Sunflower.

KWONG ON LONG CO., 686 North Spring St., Los Angeles, Calif. 90012. Mail order soy and mung beans.

RIGGSCRAFT, P.O. Box 1273, Laramie, Wyoming 82070. Shippers of sprout-quality seeds, beans and grains. Free catalogue.

NATURAL DEVELOPMENT CO., Bainbridge, Pa. 17502. Cress seeds, sunflower seeds, buckwheat, lentils, corn, wheat, alfalfa. Free postage east of the Mississippi River. Free catalogue.

SHILOH FARMS, Rt. 59, Sulphur Springs, Ark. 72768. Ask for price lists.

BEALE'S FAMOUS PRODUCTS, Box 323, Ft. Washington, Pa. 19034. Unglazed pottery sprouter, assortment of 15 different seeds, breakfast mix, salad mix, sandwich mix, books. Send for price lists.

APHRODISIA, 28 Carmine St., New York, N.Y. 10014. Alfalfa, fenugreek, flax, black and yellow mustard seeds, safflower, sesame seeds. Catalogue.

MELLINGER'S, INC., 2310 West South Range Road, North Lima, OH 44452.

D. V. BURRELL SEED GROWERS CO., P.O. Box 150, Rocky Ford, Colorado 81067.

L. L. OLDS SEED CO., 2901 Packers Avenue, P.O. Box 1069, Madison, Wisconsin 53701.

ORGANIC FARM AND GARDEN CENTER, Box 2806, San Rafael, California 94901.

RAW OLIVE OIL

CAROTHERS BROTHERS, Box 192, Mt. Dora, Fla. 32757.

WALNUT ACRES, Penns Creek, Pa. 17862. Seeds, produce. Reasonable prices.

RIGHTWAY ENTERPRISE, 113 South B St., Poterville, Ca. 93257.

VITA GREEN FARMS, P.O. Box 878, Vista, Ca. 92083. Produce.

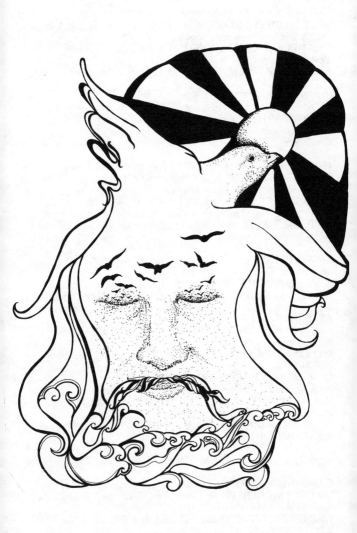

SUGGESTED READING LIST

PHYSIOLOGICAL ENIGMA OF THE WOMAN—Compilation, study of menstruation. How to overcome this disorder **$5.00**

THE SCIENCE AND PRACTICE OF IRIDOLOGY—Dr. Jensen, Study of iris for diagnosing the condition of internal organs. Study of healing crisis. Color photos. Introduction .... **50¢**
Text **$20.00**

MODERN LIVE JUICE THERAPY, Dr. Johnny Lovewisdom. Autobiography of a hermit living at 13,000 foot high Andes, who did 2 fast of over 6 month duration, each. **$1.50**

LOVEWISDOM MESSAGE ON PARADISE BUILDING, Updated version of The History of Naturalistic Tropical Colonization, Johnny Lovewisdom **$2.00**

VITARIANISM, Spiritualized Dietetics, Dr. Johnny Lovewisdom **$5.00**

HEALTHY CHILDREN, Ann Wigmore **$2.00**

MAN'S HIGHER CONSCIOUSNESS, Prof. Hotema, Fruitarianism, Vegetarianism, Longevity, Sex, Breatharianism, Cosmic Energy **$7.00**

FOOD IS YOUR BEST MEDICINE—Dr. Bieler, M.D. **$2.00**

WHAT IS TOXEMIA?—Dr. Tilden, M.D. **$1.00**

FOOD COMBINING MADE EASY—Dr. Shelton, Study of Digestion **$1.75**

FRUIT, THE FOOD AND MEDICINE OF MAN—M. Krok **$5.00**

ESSENE GOSPEL OF PEACE—E. Szekely, Live food and living love teachings of Jesus on the healing forces of Nature **$1.00**

FIELD GUIDE TO WILD EDIBLE PLANTS—B. Angier Author of 23 books on wilderness living. Quick, easy to identify, all in color drawings of ʻ120 edible wild foods

growing free in the United States and Canada. Paperback
256 Pgs. 5½ x 8½ **$5.95**
NATURAL BIRTH CONTROL—Art Rosenblum **$3.00**
HEALTHY PETS—Dr. Wigmore, The
Vegetarian Way **$1.00**
HANDBOOK TO HIGHER CONSCIOUSNESS—Ken
Keyes Jr. One of the most important, practical books on
how to love yourself and relate lovingly to others. The
method is structured so that you can reach the higher states
while living in your everyday life. Enables you to stay high
24 hrs. a day **$3.00**
**DICK GREGORY'S NATURAL DIET FOR FOLKS
WHO EAT: COOKING WITH MOTHER NATURE**—
Dick Gregory (Harper & Row Pub., NYC) The most prac-
tical book for sane transition into a fruitarian diet. How
the body works. Pets, children. Mr. Gregory is finishing his
third year of fruit juice diet and fasting **$2.00**
BE YOUR OWN DOCTOR, Ann Wigmore, Hippocrates
Health Institute, founder **$2.00**
WHY SUFFER, Ann Wigmore, Autobiography **$3.00**
NEW AGE DIRECTORY Viktoras Kulvinskas — Over 2500 entries.
Healing — resorts, schools, study centers, workshops. The following
categories are included: Vegetarian resources; vegetarian organizations;
vegetarian magazines & research; friends of animals; vegetarian teachers; healing directories; referral services; health resorts; holistic healing
centers; fruitarian resources; suggestions for fruit festival; instant holiness
by degree; aids to the study of healing; healing study referral services;
healing study centers (live food plus, herbology, naturopathy, chiro-
practic/osteopathy; homeopathy, individuals & new groups, sex and
natural childbirth education, establishment schools, massage & energy
balance, radiation study, body tests, diagnoses); spiritual centers &
courses; services & study; New Age centers; coops and produce
organizations; seed & plant sources; fruit/vegetable/grain farms; back to
the land; community living; recreation; publishers; New Age periodicals;
scientific nutritional journals; New Age products; detoxification (cleans-
ing) products; workshops/conferences. Each entry is annotated. Indexed
on subject, state and alphabetic. The world is changing. This directory will
put you in touch with what can help you. **The most updated (6/78)
listing of raw foodist resources for services, people, communi-
ties, resorts and schools. Art by Jean White, color cover by
Denis Poitras. 140 pages, 5 by 8 in. Limited edition.** **$2.75**

OMango d'Press
P.O. Box 255SL
Wethersfield, CT 061109

SURVIVAL
INTO THE 21st CENTURY

Body Ecology, Spiritual Alchemy and
Aquarian Eugenics.
Viktoras Peter Kulvinskas, M.S. Will you be alive in
1984? 2000? 2100? Are you healthy today?

Read this manual for practical information on starting the path of natural living. Discover a healthful, youthful, spiritual, life style. Obtain organic food inexpensively. YOU CAN LIVE ON AN ALL ORGANIC FOOD DIET FOR LESS THAN $3.00 PER WEEK. Learn to recognize early warnings of impending chronic ailments, how to make a painless transition to a health-improving vegetarian diet to repair and maintain health.

This manual evaluates Kosher, vegetarian, macrobiotic, live food vegetarian, city fruitarian (SPROUTARIAN), liquitarian diet. Try a low protein, low starch, low fat, low mineral, high vitamin, high enzyme, live food diet for vitality, health, strength, endurance, regeneration, spirituality. Create a natural-normal child —a genious housed in a body of health and beauty.

How to become a Naturopath doctor (in the future there will be no need for this discipline—all will be beautiful and health); diagnosis, physiognomy, iridology, acupressure. Elimination of menstruation and menopause; continence; function of sex; breast-feeding; cause and elimination of cancer, diabetes, arthritis, hypoglycemia, szhizophrenia.

WHEATGRASS THERAPY for rejuvenation, correction of chronic ailments. WATER FAST for purification, heightened awareness, spiritual adventure. INDOOR ORGANIC GARDENING—grow all your food indoors in 7 days. SPROUTING—grow a complete meal in a jar, requiring only daily watering—one pound of seed produces seven pounds of sprouts. Prepare for FAMINE, STRIKES, REVOLUTION.

TASTY RECIPES arranged in health-promoting combinations. ACUPRESSURE (pressure message of feet)—for immediate relief of headache, constipation, dizziness. Complete loving body MASSAGE.

The processes of disease, NATURAL HEALING, fasting discussed

149

at the cellular level for clear understanding of how disease is created and health regained. Appendix gives addresses for shopping by mail, health resorts, communes, New Age schools, directory of directories, reading list for continuing education.

Tropical colonization; grasss and sprouts for city survival; weed hunting and illustrations; food storage; selective non-organic food shopping. Build a $12 distiller, up to 4 gallons a day. Start an inexpensive organic restaurant.

Sunshine for lunch—breatharianiam; The temple of God and the river of Life; Cosmic forces of light and color therapy; Fruitarian aura; Nature of God; Structure of the Universe; The path of Yoga; Meditation; Karma; Reincarnation; Soul life.

The book reaches the inner person on the level of simplicity. IT IS THE FIRST REAL CHALLENGE AND AN ALTERNATIVE TO THE MACROBIOTIC. The book represents 4 years of preparation, which involved 2 years background study at Harvard Medical Library, self experimentation, plus observing the consequences and rejuvenation of others while acting as dietary "guru."

The book contains over 300 medical journal references. The appendix includes in excess of the following list of resources: 140 sources for seeds and fruit; 70 healing schools; 80 new age centers; 70 vegetarian activist groups; 250 books and reviews.

The first printing of Survival appeared Sept. 1975. The introduction is by Dick Gregory. Full color cover by Peter Max—the arrival of a cosmic being to the virgin planet earth. The back cover is by Jean Whtie—the return to the Garden of Eden. She has included over 50 most beautiful visions, as well as many scientifically accurate physiological illustrations. Many photos of transformations. The text is 320 pages, 8 by 11, perfect bound paperback $8.00.

NEW AGE RESOURCES

An extensive 32 page, 8 by 11, release has been prepared which contains some of the artwork, as well as the cover, introduction, table of content, excerpts and reviews. Plus another 10 page writeup on books of longevity, sex, fruitarianism, live foods, esoteric, new age material. Send 50¢.

LOVE YOUR BODY—A RECIPE
BY VIKTORAS KULVINSKAS

The greatest minds of all ages have been of one accord that love is the most important and powerful word in any language. We are now learning that any thing that is the recipient of the high vibrations of love flourishes and expands to the very ultimate of its potential for good. It is impossible to love your body in the highest sense and transgress nature's laws concerning it at the same time.

The book deals exclusively with the deepest truths concerning these laws. It dips into antiquity for its material and at the same time presses forward into hitherto unexplored areas in the way of original ideas and recipes, based on living food program.

Although perfect health and happiness through the use of correct nourishment is the main theme of the book, other aspects of the body care are not neglected as we learn that every part of our being unifies with the whole, even as each one of us seeks to unify with the greater whole . . . the universe. Love is the great unifier.

Love your body the live food organic way. We can treat ourselves with love and become more healthy and more beautiful. Through right diet, we can slim the body, rejuvenate it, make it youthful. Children born from such parents will now endless youth, beauty and total freedom from disease. They will love everybody. The REJUVENATING properties of these recipes—high vitamin, high enzyme, high quality protein, low calorie, mucuslean, low fat, alkalizing, natural LAETRILE (anti-cancer vitamin)—makes it an ideal diet for those who wish to overcome arthritis, rheumatism, cancer, heart disorders, obesity, aging, schizophrenia.

* Over 200 recipes of raw and cooked food, all from nonanimal sources, for transition to New Age diet.

* Recipes utilize available health foods. Prepare exotic meals in 10 to 30 minutes for up to 25, and more people.

* Over 20 pages of basic concepts of natural nutrition. Takes the confusion out of healthy diet. Makes it easy to stay young and vital.

* Recipes include many micronutrients that are absolutely essen-

151

tial for protection against smog. The diet creates pollution free body ecology.

* GOOD FOOD COMBINATIONS for easy digestion, color, loving disposition and consciousness expension.
* CHEESES FROM SEEDS. Ready in 12 hours. No culture needed. All raw, high enzyme, easily digestible. Discover in seeds a natural, untreated cheese, yogurt and milk.
* The recipes use fruit, vegetable, seed, grain, nuts, sprouts, indoor greens, weeds, oil and spices to produce varied delightful meals.
* The diet slims you down with increased vitality.
* LIVE ORGANICALLY ON LESS THAN $2/WEEK. Original complete diet at a cost of 2 cents PER MEAL.
* Grow indoors organic FOUNTAIN OF YOUTH DRINK in 7 days at cost of 10 per quart. Sweeter than all nature's nectars. Rejuvenating.

This recipe book is right for our synthetic unnatural age. It is written for survival. There are many books on the market filled with recipes heavenly in the mouth and hell in the stomach. My emphasis is upon preparing, from live food, tasty, simple, colorful combinations in harmony with the physiological limitations of the body. $2.50

Author foresees a time when we will all be living in sunshine, love and eating from our own orchards. The smiling fruitarians will once again be the guru-priests, scientists to lead humanity back to god consciousness and joyful living.

The author was sick most of his life. At an early age was semi-conscious for many weeks from typhoid fever. By the age 29, he had suffered many years from ulcer, migraine, insomnia, acne, constipation, receding hairline and graying hair. His recovery to health centered on live food, juices, sprouts as well as rediscovery of a positive feeling toward self and others. In order to devote the time to helping others and study natural healing, he left behind the teaching of math (U-Conn) and computer programming. For over 7 years, he has participated in many capacities at the Hippocrates Health Institute, which included gardening, custodian service, research, lecturing, promotion, writing, publishing, as well as acting during the last few years as co-director. In 1975, he was invited to be a guest speaker at the World Vegetarian Conference, U-Maine.

LIGHT
EATING FOR SURVIVAL

BY MARCIA ACCIARDO
Introduction by Swami Satchidanandaji Maharaj
Art by Peter Max
Preface by Viktoras Kulvinskas

NO MEAT, FISH, EGGS, OR DAIRY HERE!
RECIPES FROM

Flowers
Weeds
Sprouts
Indoor Greens
Nuts
Sea Weeds
Seeds
Grains
Herbs
Spices
Olive Oil
Yeast
Dehydrates
Algae
Vegetables
Fruit
..And lots of
LOVE

OVER 450 RAW FOOD RECIPES FOR:

Appetizers
Breads, Butters
Cakes, Croquettes, Candy
Cereals, Cheese, cookies
Drinks, Dips, Dressings
Eggnog
Juices from Grasses, Sprouts,
   Fruits, Weeds & Vegetables
Ketchup
Liver flushes, Loaves
Mayonnaise, Milks, Marinade
Nut Creams
Pizza, Puddings
Soups, Spreads, Suncheeses
Sauerkrouts, Sauces
Taco, Tofu
Yogurt

6"x9", 112 Pages
SPIRAL–BOUND

$5.95

Marcia Acciardo, Virgo, Age 21, has been a vegetarian for 8 years. She managed and was the cook of New Age Restaurant in Portland, Me. She is an experienced caterer for vegetarian functions and conferences, and spends a large amount of time traveling and giving workshops.

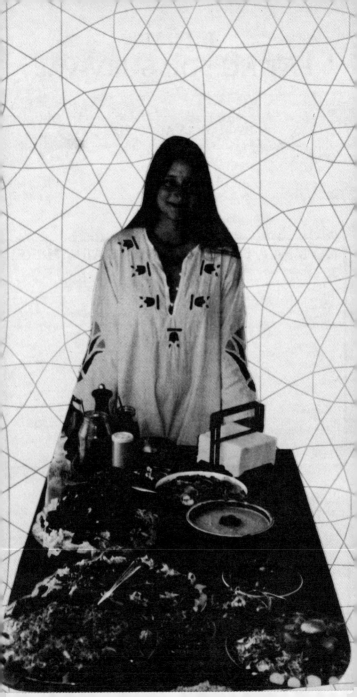

“ I have long felt the need for a live food book which can satisfy the health–conscious public that is looking for a tasty way to make a change into the New Age , low–stress diet based on nature's predigested vegetarian foods.

Marcia Acciardo's book, LIGHT EATING FOR SURVIVAL, exceeds my highest expectations. I witnessed her magic performances in many salad bars as she transformed a few simple ingredients into a melody of rainbow colors, heightened by herbal fragrance, which delighted the palate and provided optimal nutrition.

I was so pleased when she decided to share this magic in her new book. Her preparations make it easy to substitute natural foods without having the shock of sensory withdrawal while giving up the overspiced, processed dead foods. **Her attitude is "Let the sun do the cooking in the fields, while we use the stove sparingly."**

We are living in an age where eating lots of raw foods is essential. Cooking destroys many of the vitamins, all of the enzymes, chelated minerals, nucleic acids and chlorophyll. The heat disorganizes the protein structure, leading to deficiency of some of the essential amino acids. The lack of complete protein in the diet contributes to premature aging. If the diet is at least 80% raw this does not occur.

Researchers all over the world are showing that **the body is self healing when it is nourished on living foods and fresh juices.** **”**

...Viktoras Kulvinskas

**Shattered disk,
paralysis,
surgery is
followed by
grass juice fast
sprouts and
complete recovery
with love.**

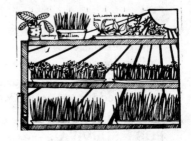

Dear Viktoras,

I just completed a 43-day fast in the desert. I've been eating sprouts
and wheatgrass for 21 days and helping some interested people in the
course of transition from meat/grain diets to raw/fruit ones. I had written
to Viktoras over a year ago telling him of my paralysis and totally
non-functioning elimination system, etc. He wrote back to me suggesting
a few avenues, all of which cost money. I had none. He suggested I fast at
home, which I did then for 50 days or more, and told me I'd soon be
healing in a river of love. True, true, Brothers and Sisters! Last Sept. 2, I
had spinal surgery to remove bone chips from inside my spinal column,
which were severing my motor nerve and causing great trauma to the
sensory nerves. The 4th lumbar vertebra was shaved down, since a bony
tumor or deposit had collected there and was blocking off all functions in
the area. The shattered disc was removed, which took the pressure off the
sciatic nerve and straightened my spine, which was slanting crazily,
anteriorly toward the right in the sacral caudal region.

I was advised after surgery of all the things I could never do again. I
lived in a hospital bed for about 2 more months doing the most shallow
breathing exercises, mental hatha yoga and meditation. By February I
was on my way to the Anza Borrega desert, where I walked, with an angel
brother who helped me, for 3 days to an isolated spot and fasted. I walked
out strong and supple after 43 days of camping above the ½-mile long
staircase of the enchanted tiger, by the river of love.

Today I begin a new 50-day fast and I am well, perfectly so. Thanks for
your real and gentle encouragement, Viktoras, when it was coming from
nowhere else but inside me and needed reinforcement. One ashram I
wrote to ask permission to fast there had told me they couldn't handle the
intensity of a person fasting as I had described, among them, etc. Some
were derisive around me, so . . . I'm able to do mayurasana again for 2
mins. and salabhasana for 60 seconds and other hatha yoga asanas, e.g.,
Ardhamatsyendrasana. I can grab and hold the opposite ankle com-
fortably indefinitely. I was told I'd never do these anymore. By now I
should be able to be painfully carefully lift a few lbs. In the desert I had to
carry 80 and 90 lb. rocks to put inside my tent to fasten it down in the 100
mph winds . . . even handstands. Surgeons' knives can't touch chatras.

Know what my cats love sprouts and eat my wheatgrass pulp every
day. When available they love watermelon pulp.

Maureen Madden